Chair Yoga for Seniors Over 60

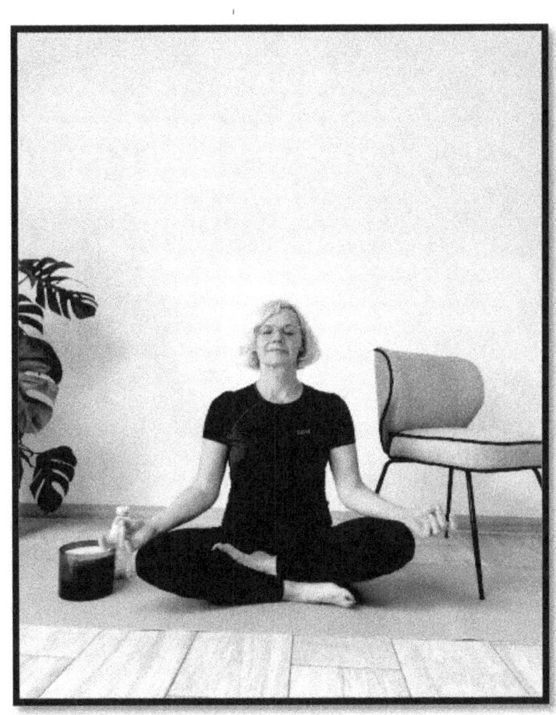

Easy-to-Follow 10 Minutes a Day Exercises and Tips for More Mobility and Boost Energy. Stay Active and Healthy, Reclaim Your Independence and Quality of Life.

Ellie Grace Rivers

Copyright Notice

Table of Contents

Disclaimer

The information provided in this book is intended for general informational purposes only. The author and publisher of this book are not licensed medical professionals, and the content of this book should not be construed as a substitute for professional medical advice. Diagnoses and treatments should only be discussed with your physician. For questions regarding a medical condition, always consult your doctor or another qualified healthcare provider.

The exercises, techniques, and advice presented in this book are intended as a general guide for Chair Yoga and should be performed with caution and under the guidance of a qualified healthcare provider. Individuals with pre-existing conditions, injuries, or physical limitations should consult their doctor before attempting the exercises or practices described in this book.

The author and publisher of this book assume no responsibility or liability for injuries, losses, or damages that may result from the use of the information contained in this book. The reader assumes full responsibility for their health and well-being, and should follow the recommendations in this book to the best of their knowledge and ability.

It is important to remember that individual results and the effectiveness of Chair Yoga exercises depend on many factors, such as a person's physical condition and consistency in practice. By reading this book, you acknowledge and agree to the terms of this disclaimer. If you do not agree with the terms of this disclaimer, please do not use the information provided in this book.

PART 1

Introduction

Welcome to the world of Chair Yoga, a gentle yet transformative practice designed specifically for seniors over 60. In our journey through life, maintaining vitality and well-being becomes increasingly essential, and yoga offers a path to achieve just that. However, traditional yoga postures might seem daunting or inaccessible to some seniors due to physical limitations or concerns about balance and flexibility. That's where Chair Yoga steps in, offering a modified approach that makes yoga accessible to everyone, regardless of age or physical condition.

In this guide, we embark on a journey to explore the enriching benefits of Chair Yoga tailored for seniors. Whether you're a seasoned yogi or new to the practice, Chair Yoga provides a safe and supportive environment to enhance your physical health, mental clarity, and emotional well-being. By harnessing the power of breath, movement, and mindfulness, Chair Yoga empowers seniors to cultivate strength, flexibility, and inner peace from the comfort of their chair.

Throughout these pages, we'll delve into a variety of Chair Yoga poses and sequences carefully crafted to address common concerns faced by seniors, such as improving posture, relieving joint stiffness, and reducing stress. Additionally, we'll explore the profound connection between mind and body, discovering how the practice of Chair Yoga can foster greater resilience, self-awareness, and a sense of vitality in our golden years.

Whether you're looking to maintain your independence, alleviate chronic pain, or simply nurture a deeper sense of well-being, Chair Yoga offers a holistic approach to aging gracefully and embracing life with renewed vitality. So, let's embark on this journey together, as we explore the transformative power of Chair Yoga for seniors over 60.

What is Yoga and it´s History?

Yoga is like a magical journey for your body, mind, and soul. It's not just stretching or bending; it's about finding harmony within yourself.

Yoga is an ancient practice that originated in India over 5,000 years ago. It encompasses a variety of physical, mental, and spiritual disciplines aimed at achieving harmony and balance in the body and mind. The word "yoga" itself means union or connection, signifying the union of the individual consciousness with the universal consciousness. Let's delve into the essence of yoga and its captivating journey through time.

Throughout history, yoga evolved and diversified into various schools and practices, each emphasizing different aspects of the discipline. From the Hatha Yoga tradition, which focuses on physical postures and breath control, to Bhakti Yoga, the path of devotion, and Jnana Yoga, the path of knowledge, there exists a yoga practice suited to every individual's temperament and spiritual aspirations.

In the late 19th and early 20th centuries, yoga gained prominence in the West, largely due to the efforts of influential figures like Swami Vivekananda and Paramahansa Yogananda, who introduced yoga philosophy and practices to Western audiences. Since then, yoga has continued to flourish globally, evolving into various styles and adaptations to meet the needs and preferences of practitioners worldwide.

Strength:

Yoga promotes flexibility and mobility through a wide range of motion exercises. Practicing yoga regularly can increase joint flexibility, reduce stiffness, and improve overall mobility, making daily activities easier and more comfortable.

Mobility:

Yoga cultivates balance through poses that challenge stability and proprioception. Standing balances like Tree Pose and Eagle Pose require focus and concentration, enhancing both physical and mental balance. Over time, consistent practice can improve balance, reducing the risk of falls and injuries, especially in older adults.

Balance:

Yoga cultivates balance through poses that challenge stability and proprioception. Standing balances like Tree Pose and Eagle Pose require focus and concentration, enhancing both physical and mental balance. Over time, consistent practice can improve balance, reducing the risk of falls and injuries, especially in older adults.

Reclaim Independence:

For individuals seeking to reclaim independence, yoga offers a gentle yet effective way to regain control over their bodies and minds. By improving strength, mobility, and balance, yoga empowers individuals to perform daily tasks with confidence and ease, fostering a sense of self-sufficiency and autonomy.

Beginners:

Yoga welcomes beginners with open arms, offering accessible classes and modifications to accommodate all levels of experience and ability. Beginners can start with basic poses and gradually progress as they build strength, flexibility, and confidence.

Boost Energy:

Yoga revitalizes the body and mind, providing a natural energy boost through mindful movement and breathwork. Dynamic sequences like Sun Salutations increase circulation, oxygenation, and energy flow throughout the body, leaving practitioners feeling invigorated and refreshed. Additionally, yoga's emphasis on relaxation and stress reduction can alleviate fatigue and restore vitality, promoting overall well-being.

In essence, yoga is a multifaceted practice that enhances strength, mobility, balance, and energy while promoting independence and well-being for practitioners of all levels. Its rich history and timeless principles continue to inspire millions worldwide to embark on a journey of self-discovery, health, and transformation.

Why Chair Yoga?

Ah, Chair Yoga—where do I even begin? It's like stumbling upon a hidden treasure in your own backyard. You see, Chair Yoga isn't just about stretching and breathing; it's about unlocking a world of possibilities right from the comfort of your favorite armchair.

Now, you might be wondering, "Why Chair Yoga?" Well, let me share with you the magic of this practice and why it holds a special place in my heart.

Accessibility is Key

One of the most beautiful aspects of Chair Yoga is its accessibility. Whether you're a sprightly senior or a busy professional with a hectic schedule, Chair Yoga welcomes you with open arms. No need to contort your body into pretzel-like poses or twist yourself into a human knot—just grab a chair and get ready to flow.

Empowering Wellness for All Ages

Chair Yoga is a practice for the people, by the people. It empowers individuals of all ages and abilities to reap the benefits of yoga, regardless of their physical limitations or mobility challenges. From improving flexibility and strength to reducing stress and enhancing balance, Chair Yoga offers a holistic approach to wellness that nourishes the body, mind, and spirit.

Gentle Yet Powerful

Don't let the word "chair" fool you—Chair Yoga packs a powerful punch. With gentle movements, mindful breathing, and a sprinkle of laughter, Chair Yoga helps you tap into your inner strength and resilience. It's about meeting yourself where you are, embracing your unique journey, and celebrating the beauty of movement in all its forms.

A Sanctuary of Solace

In today's fast-paced world, finding moments of stillness can feel like a rare luxury. But fear not, my fellow seekers of serenity, for Chair Yoga offers a sanctuary of solace in the midst of life's chaos. Whether you're craving a moment of peace amidst a busy day or seeking refuge from the storm of stress, Chair Yoga invites you to slow down, breathe deeply, and find stillness in motion.

So, my dear reader, if you're ready to embark on a journey of self-discovery, healing, and transformation, I invite you to pull up a chair and join me on the mat. Together, let's explore the boundless possibilities of Chair Yoga and unlock the door to a life filled with vitality, joy, and well-being.

Benefits of Chair Yoga for Seniors.

Now, let's explore the myriad benefits that Chair Yoga offers to seniors, empowering them to lead vibrant, healthy, and fulfilling lives.

Enhanced Flexibility and Mobility

One of the most noticeable benefits of Chair Yoga for seniors is improved flexibility and mobility. As we age, our muscles tend to become tighter, and our joints may stiffen, leading to decreased range of motion and mobility. Chair Yoga offers gentle stretching exercises that help to loosen tight muscles, lubricate the joints, and improve flexibility. With regular practice, seniors can experience greater freedom of movement and ease in daily activities such as walking, bending, and reaching.

Increased Strength and Stability

Chair Yoga isn't just about stretching—it also helps to build strength and stability, essential for maintaining independence and preventing falls as we age. Through a series of seated and standing poses, Chair Yoga strengthens the muscles of the legs, core, and upper body, improving balance and stability. Stronger muscles help seniors perform daily tasks with greater ease, reduce the risk of injury, and enhance overall quality of life.

Improved Posture and Alignment

Poor posture is common among seniors, often leading to discomfort, pain, and decreased mobility. Chair Yoga focuses on proper alignment and posture, helping seniors develop an awareness of their body's position and movement patterns. By practicing gentle spinal twists, backbends, and shoulder openers, seniors can improve their posture, alleviate tension in the muscles, and reduce the risk of chronic pain and injury.

Pain Management

Chair yoga can be an effective tool for managing chronic pain, such as arthritis or back pain. The gentle movements and stretches help to increase circulation, reduce inflammation, and alleviate muscle tension, leading to decreased pain and improved comfort.

Stress Reduction and Relaxation

In today's fast-paced world, stress has become a ubiquitous part of life, taking a toll on our physical and mental well-being. Chair Yoga offers seniors a sanctuary of peace and tranquility amidst the chaos of daily life. Through mindful breathing techniques, guided relaxation, and meditation, Chair Yoga helps seniors reduce stress, calm the mind, and cultivate a sense of inner peace and serenity. By incorporating relaxation practices into their daily routine, seniors can improve sleep quality, boost mood, and enhance overall quality of life.

Enhanced Mental Clarity and Focus

As we age, cognitive function may decline, leading to memory loss, difficulty concentrating, and mental fog. Chair Yoga offers seniors a gentle yet effective way to sharpen their mental faculties and enhance cognitive function. By engaging in mindful movement and breath awareness practices, seniors can improve mental clarity, focus, and concentration. Additionally, Chair Yoga offers opportunities for creativity, problem-solving, and self-expression, stimulating the brain and promoting overall cognitive health.

Social Connection and Community

Chair Yoga isn't just about individual practice—it's also about building connections and fostering a sense of community. Seniors who participate in Chair Yoga classes have the opportunity to connect with like-minded individuals, share experiences, and support each other on their wellness journey. The sense of camaraderie and belonging that comes from practicing yoga together can have a profound impact on seniors' emotional well-being, reducing feelings of loneliness and isolation and enhancing overall quality of life.

In conclusion, Chair Yoga offers seniors a wealth of physical, mental, and emotional benefits, empowering them to live life to the fullest. Whether you're looking to improve flexibility, strength, balance, or simply find a moment of peace in a hectic world, Chair Yoga has something to offer everyone. So, grab a chair, take a seat, and embark on a journey of health, happiness, and vitality through the transformative practice of Chair Yoga.

Namaste.

Myths and Mistakes

As we delve deeper into the practice of Chair Yoga, it's important to address common myths and potential mistakes that seniors may encounter. By debunking misconceptions and providing safety tips and modifications, we can ensure that seniors have a safe, effective, and enjoyable yoga experience.

Myth: Yoga is only for the young and flexible.

Fact: Yoga is a practice that is truly for everyone, regardless of age, fitness level, or flexibility. While it's true that mainstream yoga classes often feature young, athletic practitioners performing advanced poses, Chair Yoga offers a more accessible and inclusive approach. With the support of a chair, seniors can participate in yoga classes and reap the benefits of the practice without having to worry about performing challenging poses or contorting their bodies into pretzel-like shapes.

In fact, Chair Yoga is specifically designed to accommodate individuals with limited mobility, chronic pain, or other physical challenges. By focusing on gentle movements, breath awareness, and relaxation techniques, Chair Yoga promotes overall well-being and vitality for seniors of all abilities.

Myth: You have to be able to touch your toes to practice yoga.

Fact: Contrary to popular belief, yoga is not about achieving extreme flexibility or mastering advanced poses. At its core, yoga is about connecting with your breath, moving mindfully, and cultivating a sense of inner peace and balance. Chair Yoga embraces this philosophy by offering a variety of seated and standing poses that can be modified to accommodate seniors of all flexibility levels.

Whether you can touch your toes or not is irrelevant in Chair Yoga—the practice is about meeting yourself where you are and honoring your body's unique needs and limitations.

Myth: Chair Yoga is too easy to be effective.

Fact: While Chair Yoga may appear gentle on the surface, it can be surprisingly challenging and effective, especially for seniors who may have limited mobility or physical strength. Chair Yoga offers a holistic approach to wellness that addresses the body, mind, and spirit, incorporating elements of strength, flexibility, balance, and relaxation.

Through a combination of gentle stretching, strength-building exercises, and breath awareness practices, Chair Yoga helps seniors improve their physical health, reduce stress, and enhance their overall quality of life. Plus, Chair Yoga can be tailored to suit individual needs and preferences, making it accessible and enjoyable for seniors of all fitness levels.

Myth: You need special equipment to practice Chair Yoga.

Fact: One of the great things about Chair Yoga is its simplicity and accessibility—all you need is a sturdy chair with a straight back and armrests to get started. While optional props such as yoga mats, cushions, and straps can enhance your practice, they are not necessary to experience the benefits of Chair Yoga.

In fact, many Chair Yoga poses can be modified using items commonly found around the house, such as towels, pillows, and belts. The key is to adapt the practice to suit your individual needs and preferences, making it accessible and enjoyable for seniors of all walks of life.

Safety Tips and Modifications:

1. **Listen to your body:** Pay attention to how your body feels during practice and honor your limitations. If a pose causes pain or discomfort, back off and modify as needed. Remember, yoga is not about pushing yourself to the point of strain or injury—it's about finding ease and comfort in each pose.

2. **Use props for support:** Chairs, cushions, and blankets can provide support and stability during Chair Yoga practice. Use props to modify poses and make them more accessible and comfortable. For example, placing a cushion under your seat can provide extra support for your hips and lower back, while using a chair for balance can help you maintain stability during standing poses.

3. **Practice mindfulness:** Stay present and mindful throughout your practice, focusing on your breath and body sensations. Avoid pushing yourself beyond your limits and practice self-compassion and acceptance. Remember, Chair Yoga is not a competition—it's a journey of self-discovery and self-care.

4. **Communicate with your teacher:** If you're attending a Chair Yoga class, don't hesitate to communicate with your teacher about any concerns, injuries, or limitations you may have. Your teacher can offer modifications and adjustments to ensure a safe and enjoyable practice. Plus, they can guide proper alignment and technique to help you get the most out of your practice.

5. **Stay hydrated:** Drink plenty of water before, during, and after your Chair Yoga practice to stay hydrated and support your body's natural detoxification processes. Hydration is key to maintaining energy levels, promoting healthy circulation, and supporting overall well-being.

By dispelling myths, addressing potential mistakes, and implementing safety tips and modifications, seniors can enjoy a safe, effective, and enjoyable Chair Yoga practice that promotes health, happiness, and well-being. With patience, persistence, and a sense of curiosity, Chair Yoga can become a valuable tool for seniors to enhance their physical health, reduce stress, and cultivate a deeper sense of connection with themselves and the world around them.

Everybody is Different

The exercises detailed in the upcoming chapters cater to individuals of all backgrounds, whether you've been dedicated to fitness for years or if gym visits are a distant memory. These routines are crafted to be straightforward, accessible, and notably impactful. Remember to pace yourself. There's no rush to attempt all exercises on the initial day. Each person will have varying comfort levels with movement and exertion. Furthermore, these thresholds may fluctuate daily. You might breeze through several exercises today but find yourself inclined towards just a couple tomorrow.

Your body communicates through unmistakable signals when something isn't right. Experiencing dizziness or light-headedness, for instance, serves as a clear indication to pause or cease activity. While mild discomfort during exercise and subsequent soreness are common, sharp or enduring pain signifies a need to halt.

Lastly, allow yourself adequate rest. Although integrating movement into daily life is beneficial, rigorous workouts every day aren't advisable. Allocate one to two days weekly for recovery. On these rest days, engage in gentle activities like walking, swimming, or dancing to keep your body mobile without pushing it to its limits.

PART 2

Getting Ready for Chair Yoga

Now that we've explored the foundational aspects of Chair Yoga, let's dive into the practical steps for getting started with your practice. From setting up your yoga space to preparing your mind and body for the journey ahead, this section will guide you through the essential elements of getting ready for Chair Yoga.

Essential Equipment

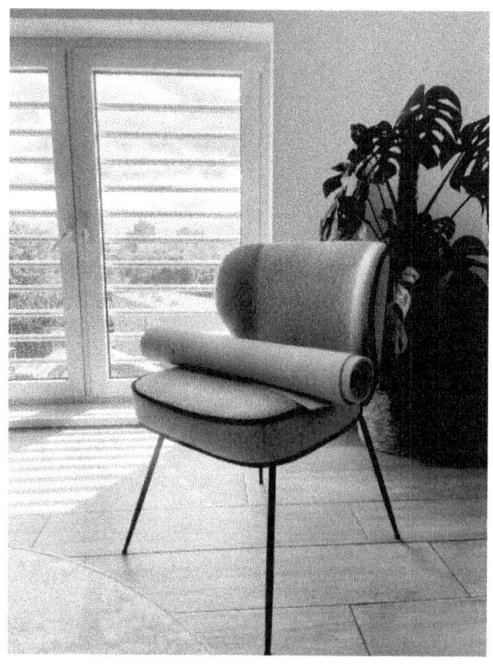

Now that we've created a comfortable and inviting space for Chair Yoga practice, let's focus on the essential equipment that will help you make the most of your practice.

Sturdy Chair

One of the key elements of Chair Yoga is a sturdy and stable chair. Choose a chair with a straight back and armrests that will provide reliable support during your practice. Ensure that the chair is comfortable and safe for you, and that it does not slip or wobble during movements.

Yoga Mat

While Chair Yoga predominantly involves seated or standing poses, some exercises may require the use of a yoga mat for additional support and comfort. Choose a mat with sufficient cushioning to protect your joints and spine from impacts and discomfort during practice.

Cushions and Blankets

Cushions and blankets can be useful props for Chair Yoga, especially when performing seated poses or for support during relaxation and meditation. Place cushions under your feet or buttocks to provide additional support and comfort during practice. Blankets can be used for warmth and coziness during relaxation exercises.

Straps and Blocks

While most Chair Yoga poses do not require the use of straps and blocks, they can be helpful props for performing certain exercises and deepening your practice. Straps can help you achieve certain poses when flexibility or strength allows you to reach only to a certain extent. Blocks can be used to extend the range of motion, improve alignment, and provide additional support in challenging poses.

Reliable Timer

While not mandatory, a reliable timer can be a useful tool for Chair Yoga practice. Use a timer to measure the time for each pose or exercise, ensuring a consistent and balanced distribution of time between different aspects of your practice.

Once you've prepared the necessary equipment, you'll be ready to make the most of your Chair Yoga practice. Remember, the goal of practice is not perfection, but the process of exploring your body, mind, and soul through movement and breath.

Make Your Chair Yoga Area Comfortable

Creating a comfortable environment for your Chair Yoga practice is essential to enhance your experience and maximize the benefits of the practice. Here are some tips to help you make your Chair Yoga area as cozy and inviting as possible:

1. **Clear Clutter:** Start by clearing any clutter or distractions from your practice area. A tidy space helps create a sense of calm and allows you to focus fully on your practice without unnecessary distractions.

2. **Choose a Quiet Space:** Select a quiet and peaceful area in your home where you can practice without interruptions. Ideally, choose a space with minimal noise and distractions to create a serene environment for your practice.

3. **Set the Mood:** Consider setting the mood with soft lighting, calming music, or scented candles to create a relaxing atmosphere. You can also incorporate elements like plants or artwork that inspire and uplift you, making your practice space feel more personal and inviting.

4. **Adjust the Temperature:** Make sure the temperature in your practice area is comfortable and conducive to relaxation. You may want to adjust the thermostat or use blankets or layers to ensure you stay warm during your practice.

5. **Use Comfortable Props:** Gather any props or accessories you may need for your practice, such as cushions, blankets, or bolsters. These props can provide additional support and comfort during your practice, allowing you to relax more deeply into each pose.

6. **Personalize Your Space:** Add personal touches to your practice area that resonate with you, such as photos, inspirational quotes, or meaningful objects. Surrounding yourself with items that bring you joy and comfort can help create a sense of sanctuary in your practice space.

By taking the time to create a comfortable and welcoming environment for your Chair Yoga practice, you can enhance your overall experience and cultivate a deeper sense of relaxation and well-being. Remember that your practice area is your sanctuary, so make it a place where you feel calm, supported, and at peace.

Positive Mindset

Creating a positive mindset is crucial for a fulfilling Chair Yoga practice. Your mindset shapes your experience, influencing how you perceive challenges, setbacks, and successes. Here are some strategies to cultivate a positive mindset for your Chair Yoga practice:

1. **Cultivate Gratitude:** Begin your practice with a sense of gratitude for the opportunity to nourish your body, mind, and spirit through Chair Yoga. Take a moment to reflect on the things you are grateful for in your life, whether it's your health, loved ones, or the beauty of nature. Cultivating gratitude can shift your focus from what you lack to what you have, fostering a sense of abundance and contentment.

2. **Set Positive Intentions:** Before starting your practice, set positive intentions to guide your mindset and focus. Whether it's cultivating self-compassion, increasing flexibility, or finding inner peace, setting clear and positive intentions can help you stay focused and motivated throughout your practice. Repeat your intentions silently or out loud to yourself as a reminder of your goals and aspirations.

3. **Practice Self-Compassion:** Be kind and compassionate towards yourself during your Chair Yoga practice. Let go of judgment and perfectionism, and instead embrace a mindset of self-acceptance and self-love. Remember that Chair Yoga is a journey, not a destination, and it's okay to make mistakes or have setbacks along the way. Treat yourself with the same kindness and understanding you would offer to a dear friend.

4. **Focus on the Present Moment:** Anchor your awareness in the present moment during your Chair Yoga practice. Instead of dwelling on the past or worrying about the future, bring your attention to the sensations of your breath, the movements of your body, and the sounds around you. Practicing mindfulness in this way can help you cultivate a sense of peace and serenity, allowing you to fully immerse yourself in the present moment.

5. **Celebrate Your Progress:** Acknowledge and celebrate your progress, no matter how small or incremental it may seem. Whether it's mastering a new pose, deepening your breath, or experiencing moments of inner calm, take time to acknowledge and celebrate your achievements along the way. Recognizing your progress can boost your confidence and motivation, inspiring you to continue growing and evolving in your practice.

By incorporating these strategies into your Chair Yoga practice, you can cultivate a positive mindset that supports your overall well-being and growth. Remember that your mindset is a powerful tool that can shape your experience, so choose to approach your practice with positivity, openness, and self-compassion.

Health Expert

Consulting with your healthcare expert is a pivotal step when considering the integration of Chair Yoga into your wellness routine. This proactive approach ensures that you embark on your yoga journey with a clear understanding of how it aligns with your individual health needs and goals. Let's delve deeper into the importance of consulting with your healthcare provider before delving into Chair Yoga practice.

First and foremost, consulting with your healthcare expert allows for a comprehensive assessment of your current health status. Your healthcare provider possesses the expertise to evaluate any pre-existing medical conditions, injuries, or limitations that may impact your ability to engage in physical activity. Through this assessment, they can identify any potential contraindications or risks associated with Chair Yoga and provide tailored recommendations to ensure your safety and well-being.

Moreover, your healthcare provider can collaborate with you to develop a personalized Chair Yoga plan that meets your specific needs and goals. They can offer valuable insights into how Chair Yoga can complement your existing treatment regimen or rehabilitation program, providing a holistic approach to managing your health. By working together with your healthcare provider, you can design a practice that addresses your unique challenges and empowers you to achieve optimal health outcomes.

Another critical aspect of consulting with your healthcare expert is the management of medications and potential interactions with Chair Yoga practice. If you are taking medications for any health conditions, your healthcare provider can offer guidance on how yoga may impact their efficacy or side effects. They can help you navigate any adjustments needed to ensure the safe and effective integration of Chair Yoga into your wellness routine.

Additionally, your healthcare provider serves as a trusted resource for monitoring your progress and addressing any concerns or questions that may arise along the way. They can track changes in your health status, mobility, and overall well-being, providing valuable feedback and guidance to support your yoga journey. Regular check-ins with your healthcare provider allow for ongoing assessment and adjustment of your Chair Yoga practice, ensuring that it remains aligned with your evolving health needs.

Furthermore, consulting with your healthcare expert fosters a sense of collaboration and empowerment in managing your health. By actively involving your healthcare provider in your decision-making process, you demonstrate a commitment to prioritizing your well-being and seeking expert guidance. This collaborative approach ensures that you have access to the support and resources you need to thrive on your yoga journey.

In conclusion, consulting with your healthcare expert before embarking on Chair Yoga practice is a proactive and essential step in prioritizing your health and safety. Your healthcare provider's expertise, guidance, and support are invaluable assets as you navigate the integration of yoga into your wellness routine. By working together, you can develop a personalized Chair Yoga plan that supports your health goals and empowers you to live your best life.

PART 3

Getting Started with Breathwork and Warm-Up

Now that we've laid the foundation for your Chair Yoga practice, let's dive into the first steps of your journey: breathwork and warm-up exercises. In this section, we'll explore the importance of conscious breathing and gentle movements to prepare your body and mind for the deeper aspects of your practice.

Simple Breathing Techniques

Breathwork is a fundamental aspect of yoga, serving as a bridge between the body and mind. Conscious breathing techniques, known as pranayama, help to calm the nervous system, increase oxygen flow, and cultivate mindfulness. As we embark on this journey, let's explore some simple breathwork exercises to center and ground ourselves before moving into the physical practice.

1. **Deep Belly Breathing(Diaphragmatic Breathing):** Find a comfortable seated position in your chair, with your feet flat on the floor and your hands resting on your thighs. Close your eyes and take a few moments to connect with your breath. Place one hand on your belly and the other on your chest. Inhale deeply through your nose, allowing your belly to expand like a balloon. Exhale slowly through your mouth, drawing your navel towards your spine. Repeat this deep belly breathing for several rounds, focusing on the gentle rise and fall of your abdomen with each breath.

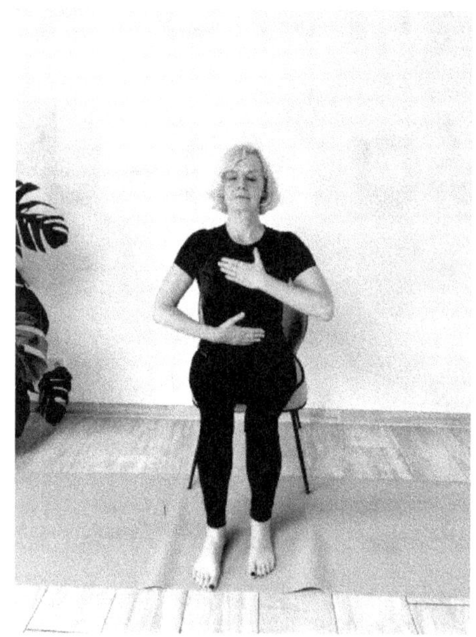

2. **Equal Ratio Breathing:** Sitting comfortably in your chair, inhale deeply through your nose for a count of four. Pause briefly at the top of your inhalation, then exhale slowly through your nose for a count of four. Continue this equal ratio breathing pattern for several rounds, maintaining a smooth and steady rhythm. As you breathe, imagine each inhale filling you with energy and vitality, while each exhale releases tension and stress from your body and mind.

3. **Alternate Nostril Breathing (Nadi Shodhana):** This ancient yogic technique balances the flow of energy in the body and calms the mind. Sit comfortably in your chair and bring your right hand to your nose. Use your right thumb to close your right nostril and your ring finger to close your left nostril. Begin by closing your right nostril and inhaling deeply through your left nostril. Then, close your left nostril and exhale completely through your right nostril. Inhale through your right nostril, then close it and exhale through your left nostril. Continue this alternate nostril breathing for several rounds, maintaining a steady and even breath.

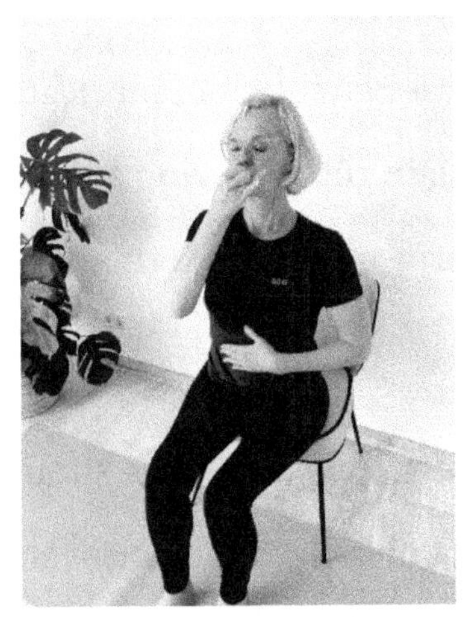 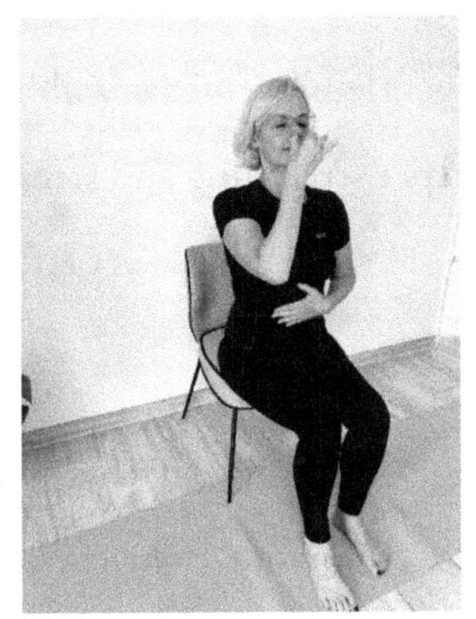 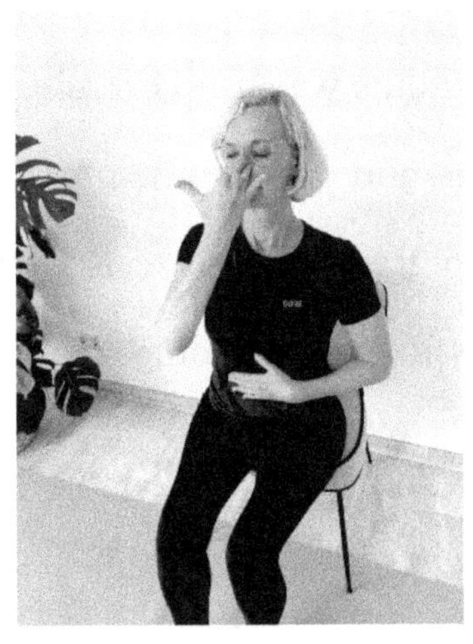

4. **Three-Part Breath (Dirga Pranayama):** Three-part breath, also known as Dirga Pranayama, is a calming and grounding breathing technique that helps to deepen the breath and expand lung capacity. To practice three-part breath, sit comfortably in your chair with your spine tall and your shoulders relaxed. Place one hand on your abdomen and the other hand on your chest. Inhale deeply through your nose, allowing your belly to expand first, then filling your chest with air, and finally allowing the breath to rise into your upper chest. Exhale slowly and completely through your nose, releasing the breath from your upper chest, then your chest, and finally allowing your belly to contract. Continue this three-part breath pattern for several rounds, feeling the breath flow smoothly and evenly throughout your entire body. As you breathe, focus on creating a sense of expansion and spaciousness within yourself, allowing each inhale to fill you with

vitality and each exhale to release any tension or stress.

After completing these breathwork exercises, take a moment to notice how you feel. Notice any shifts in your energy, mood, or awareness. Allow yourself to fully embody the present moment and the sensations in your body.

Warm-Up Exercises

Now that we've primed our bodies and minds with breathwork, it's time to gently awaken the body with some warm-up exercises. These gentle movements will help increase circulation, lubricate the joints, and prepare the muscles for deeper stretching and strengthening in the following sections of our practice. In this section, we'll explore some simple yet effective warm-up exercises that you can incorporate into your Chair Yoga routine.

1. **Neck Rolls:** Sit comfortably in your chair with your spine tall and your shoulders relaxed. Inhale as you gently drop your right ear towards your right shoulder, feeling a stretch along the left side of your neck. Exhale as you roll your chin towards your chest, then inhale as you lift your head back to center. Repeat this movement on the opposite side, rolling your left ear towards your left shoulder. Continue to alternate sides, moving with your breath and allowing your head to move in a slow and controlled manner.

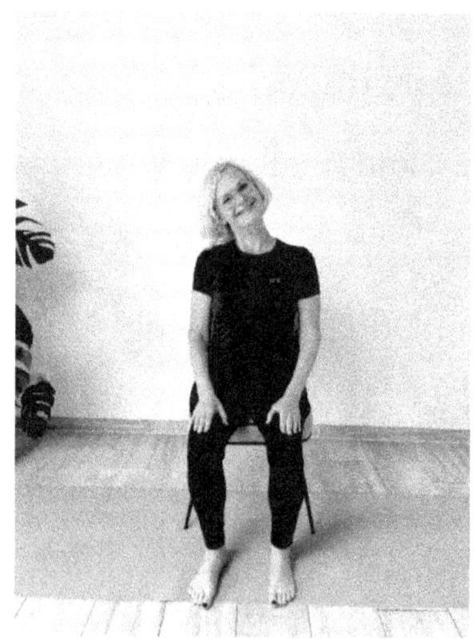
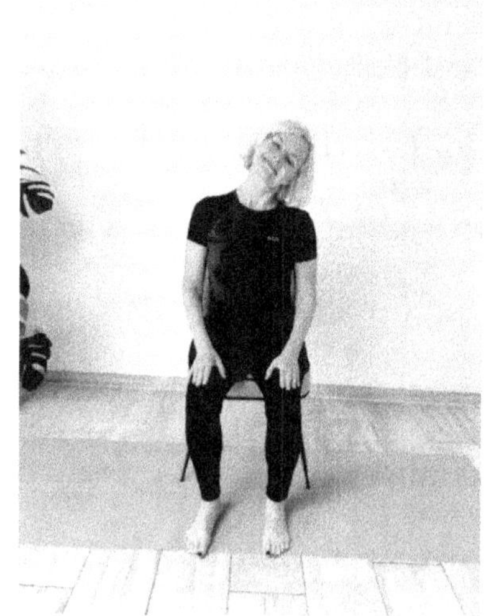

2. **Shoulder Shrugs:** Inhale as you lift your shoulders up towards your ears, feeling a gentle contraction in the muscles of your upper back. Exhale as you roll your shoulders back and down, feeling a release of tension in your shoulders and neck. Repeat this movement several times, allowing your breath to guide the motion and soften any areas of tension or tightness.

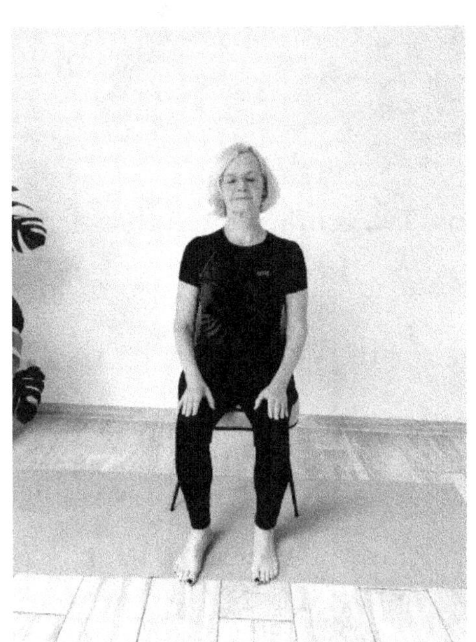
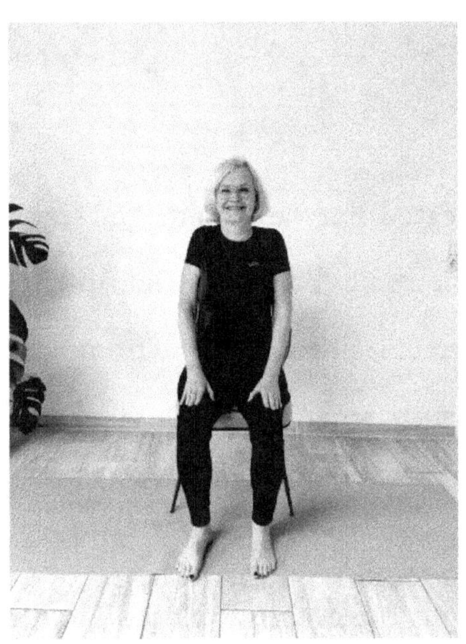

3. **Seated Cat-Cow Stretch:** Sit towards the front edge of your chair with your feet flat on the floor and your hands resting on your knees. Inhale as you arch your back and lift your chest towards the ceiling, drawing your shoulder blades together. Exhale as you round your spine and tuck your chin towards your chest, feeling a stretch along your upper back. Continue to move through these seated cat-cow stretches, flowing with your breath and exploring the full range of motion in your spine.

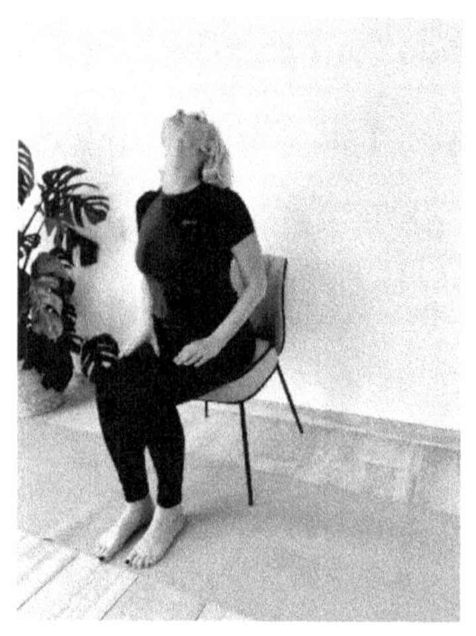
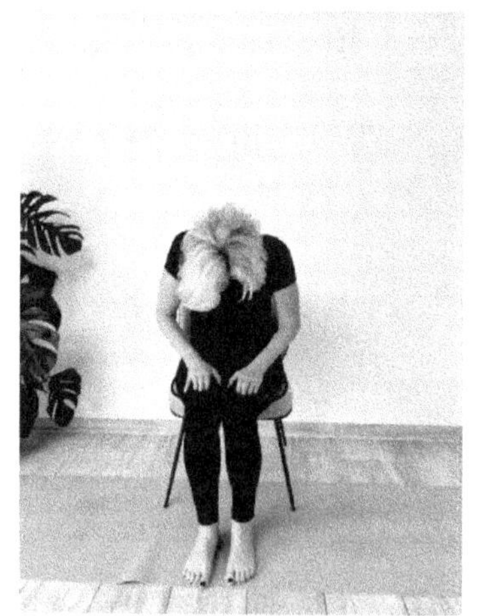
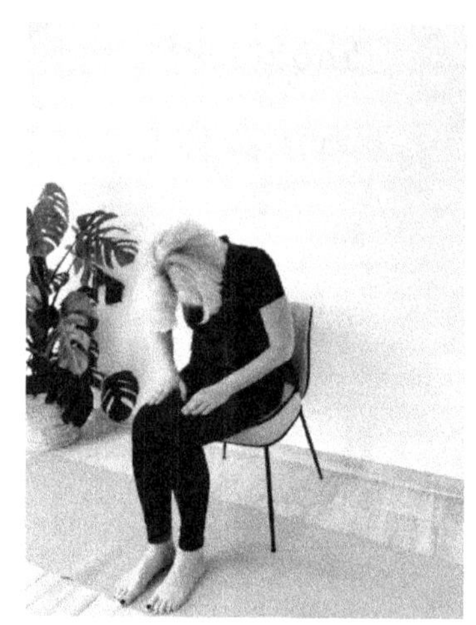

4. **Seated Forward Fold**: The seated forward fold is a gentle stretch that helps to lengthen the spine, release tension in the hamstrings, and promote relaxation. To perform this stretch, sit towards the front edge of your chair with your feet flat on the floor and your hands resting on your thighs. Inhale as you lengthen your spine and lift your chest towards the ceiling. Exhale as you hinge forward from your hips, reaching your hands towards your feet or the floor in front of you. Allow your head to hang heavy, and relax your neck and shoulders. Hold this position for a few breaths, feeling a gentle stretch along the back of your legs and spine. Then, inhale as you slowly roll back up to a seated position. As you move, focus on maintaining a smooth and steady breath, allowing each exhale to deepen the stretch.

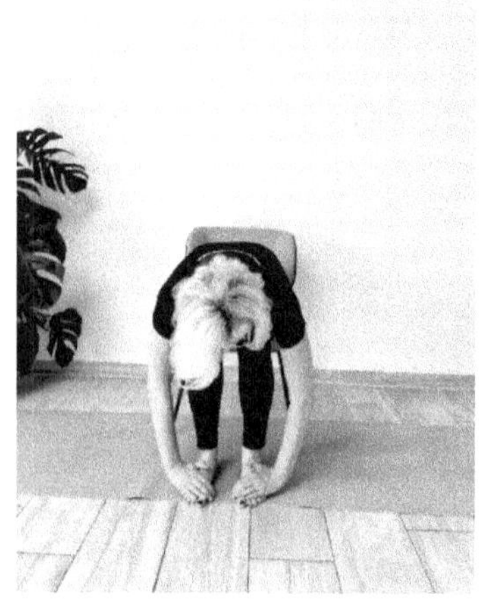
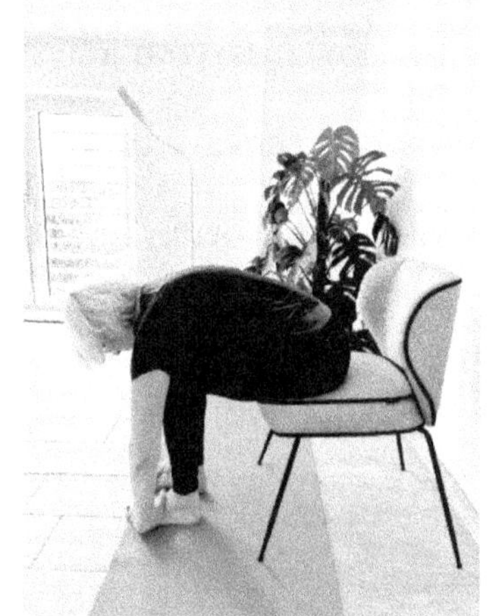
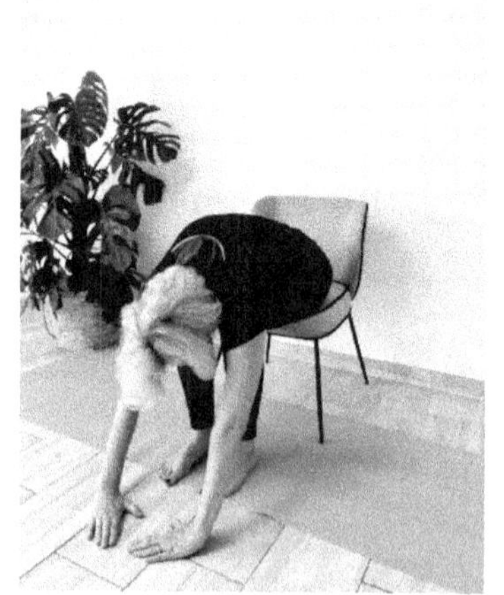

By incorporating breathwork and warm-up exercises into your Chair Yoga practice, you set a strong foundation for a safe, effective, and enjoyable experience. These gentle movements help to awaken the body, quiet the mind, and prepare you for the deeper aspects of your practice. As you continue on your Chair Yoga journey, remember to listen to your body, honor your limitations, and approach each practice with curiosity and compassion.

So, roll out your mat, take a seat in your favorite chair, and get ready to embark on a journey of self-discovery and transformation through the practice of Chair Yoga.

PART 4

Chair Yoga Basics for Beginners

In this section, we'll dive into the foundational principles of Chair Yoga, providing you with the essential tools and techniques to begin your practice with confidence and ease. Whether you're new to yoga or a seasoned practitioner looking to explore the benefits of Chair Yoga, these basics will serve as a solid foundation for your journey towards improved health and well-being.

As you begin your Chair Yoga practice, remember that it's perfectly normal to feel a bit uncertain or apprehensive at first. Give yourself permission to explore and experiment with different poses and techniques, allowing your practice to evolve and unfold naturally over time. With consistent effort and dedication, you'll gradually build strength, flexibility, and resilience, both on and off the mat.

28-Day Chair Yoga Challenge for Beginners

Dear Chair Yoga Enthusiasts, welcome to the 28-day Chair Yoga challenge for beginners! I'm delighted to have you join me on this journey towards greater health, vitality, and peace of mind. As someone who has dedicated years to practicing and teaching Chair Yoga, I understand the transformative power it holds, especially for those of us over 60.

To kickstart your journey, I've prepared seven meticulously detailed exercises that will introduce you to the fundamentals of Chair Yoga. These exercises are designed to gently stretch and strengthen your body, improve your balance, and enhance your overall well-being. But the real magic lies in the repetition.

After completing these initial exercises, I encourage you to continue practicing them daily for the next three weeks. Through repetition, you'll find that the movements become more familiar, allowing you to perform them with greater precision and ease. You'll notice subtle improvements in your strength, flexibility, and body awareness, paving the way for a stronger, fitter, and more centered version of yourself.

But Chair Yoga is not just about physical fitness—it's also about cultivating a sense of inner peace and relaxation. As you immerse yourself in these exercises, take time to connect with your breath, quiet your mind, and listen to the needs of your body. With each practice session, you'll deepen your sense of mindfulness and find yourself becoming more grounded, centered, and serene.

So, let's embark on this journey together, one breath at a time. Trust in the process, embrace the journey, and celebrate every step forward. By committing to these exercises and honoring your body's wisdom, you'll unlock a world of strength, vitality, and inner peace that will enrich every aspect of your life.

Day 1 – Day 8 – Day 15 – Day 22: Foundation Building Exercises

Building a strong foundation is essential for maintaining balance and stability in Chair Yoga practice. These foundation-building exercises focus on improving core strength, proprioception, and coordination, helping you feel more grounded and centered in your body. Incorporate these exercises into your routine to enhance your balance and overall well-being.

Start your daily Yoga Routines with Breathwork and Warm-Up Exercises.

1. **Seated Mountain Pose (Tadasana):** Sit tall in your chair with your feet flat on the floor and your spine erect. Ground down through your sit bones and imagine roots growing from your feet into the earth, anchoring you firmly in place. Engage your core muscles and lengthen your spine, reaching the crown of your head towards the ceiling. Relax your shoulders away from your ears and place your hands on your thighs or knees. Close your eyes and take a few deep breaths, feeling rooted and grounded in your seated mountain pose.

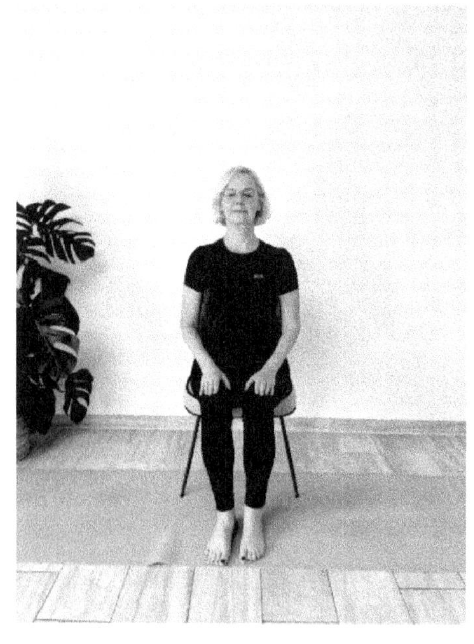 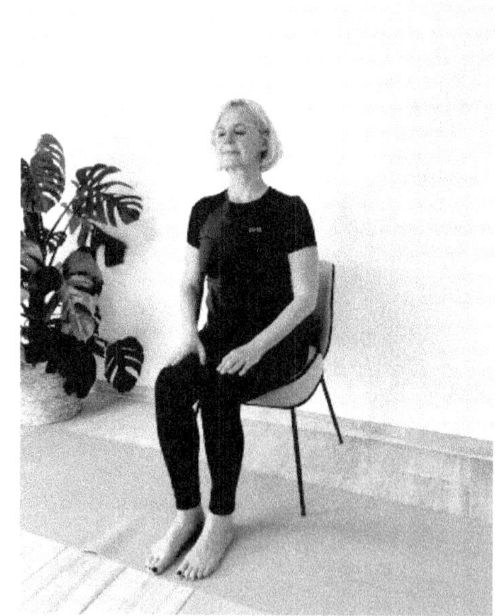

2. **Seated Tree Pose (Vrksasana):** Sit towards the front edge of your chair with your feet flat on the floor and your spine tall. Shift your weight into your right foot and lift your left foot off the floor, placing the sole of your left foot on the inside of your right calf or thigh. Press your foot into your leg and your leg into your foot, creating a firm connection between your body and the chair. Engage your core muscles and lengthen your spine, finding balance and stability in your seated tree pose. Hold for a few breaths, then switch sides.

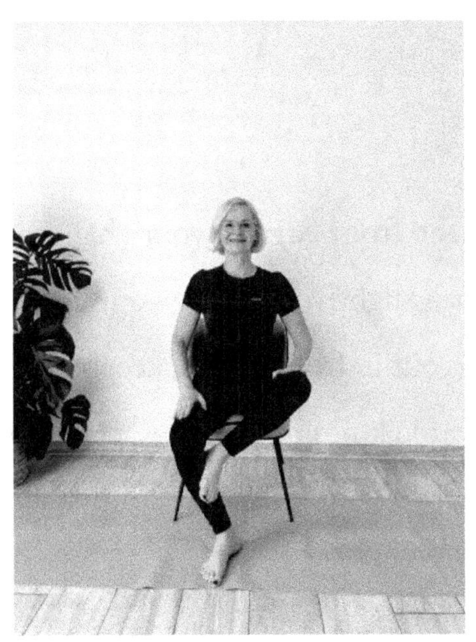 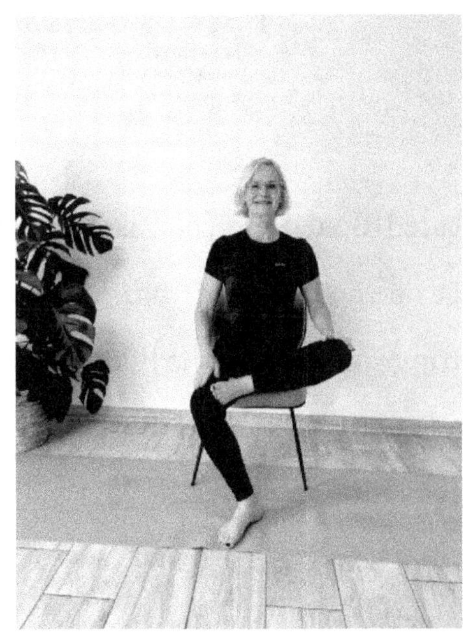

3. **Seated Warrior Pose (Virabhadrasana):** Sit towards the front edge of your chair with your feet hip-width apart and your spine tall. Extend your right leg out in front of you, bending your right knee and keeping your foot flexed. Ground down through your left foot and engage your core muscles as you reach your arms overhead, bringing your palms together. Imagine you are pressing against an invisible wall with your hands, activating your upper body and core. Hold for a few breaths, then switch sides.

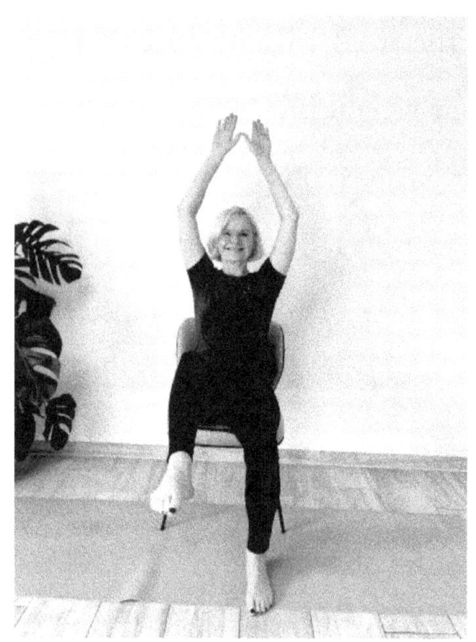
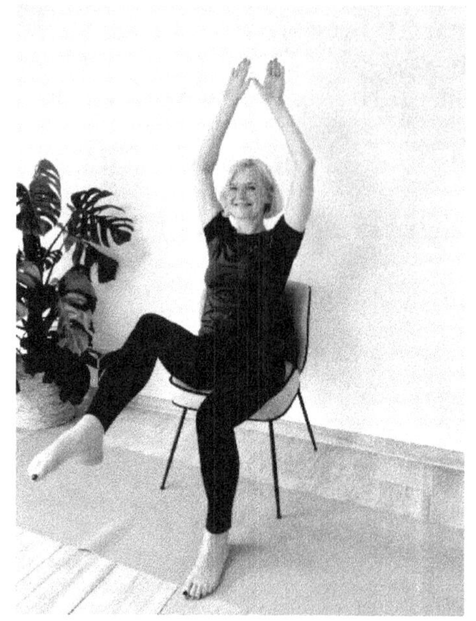

4. **Seated Boat Pose (Navasana):** Sit towards the front edge of your chair with your feet flat on the floor and your spine tall. Lean back slightly, engaging your core muscles and lifting your feet off the floor. Extend your legs out in front of you, keeping them together and your toes pointed. Reach your arms forward alongside your legs, parallel to the floor. Hold for a few breaths, engaging your core to maintain balance and stability in your seated boat pose.

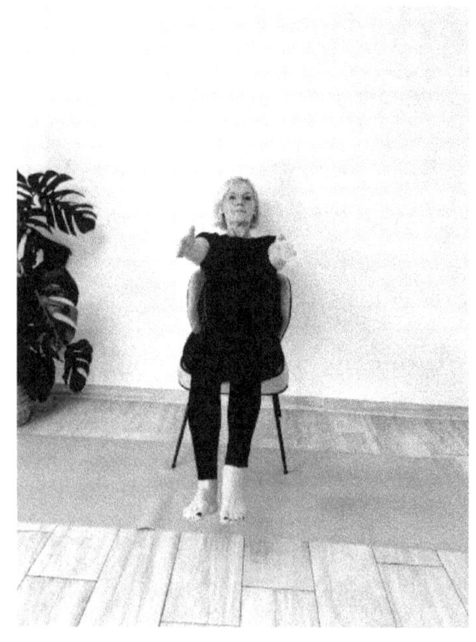
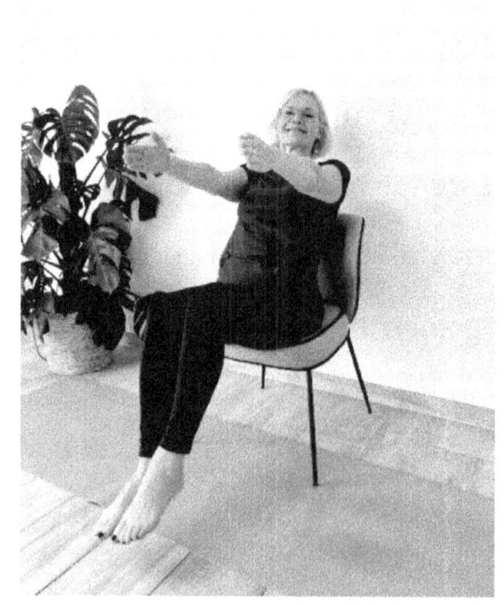

5. **Seated Side Stretch (Parsva Sukhasana):** Sit tall in your chair with your feet flat on the floor and your spine erect. Inhale as you reach your right arm up towards the ceiling, lengthening through your side body. Exhale as you gently lean to the left, stretching your right side. Keep both hips grounded on the chair and avoid collapsing into the left side. Hold for a few breaths, then switch sides.

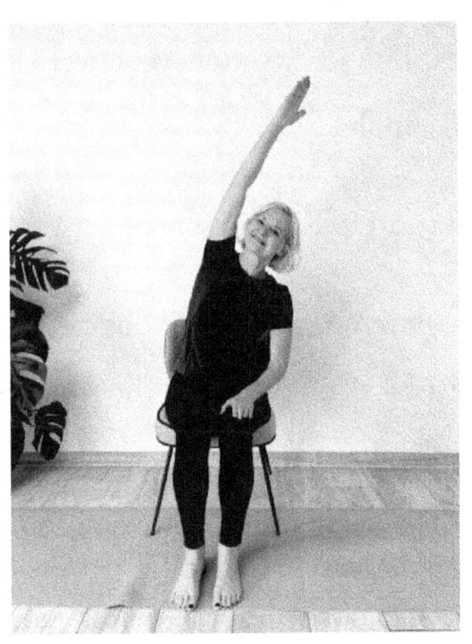 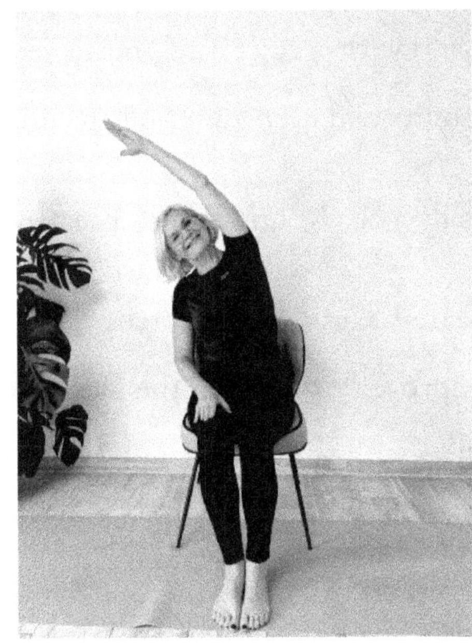

Day 2 - Day 9 – Day 16 – Day 23: Mobility Improvement

Mobility is essential for maintaining independence and quality of life as we age. Chair Yoga offers a gentle and effective way to improve mobility, flexibility, and range of motion, allowing you to move more freely and with greater ease. In this section, we'll explore some simple yet effective exercises to enhance mobility and keep your body feeling strong and supple.

Start your daily Yoga Routines with Breathwork and Warm-Up Exercises.

1. **Seated Cat-Cow Stretch:** This classic yoga stretch helps to mobilize the spine and improve flexibility in the back and torso. Start by sitting towards the front edge of your chair with your feet flat on the floor and your hands resting on your knees. Inhale as you arch your back and lift your chest towards the ceiling, drawing your shoulder blades together. Exhale as you round your spine and tuck your chin towards your chest, feeling a stretch along your upper back. Continue to move through this seated cat-cow stretch, flowing with your breath and exploring the full range of motion in your spine.

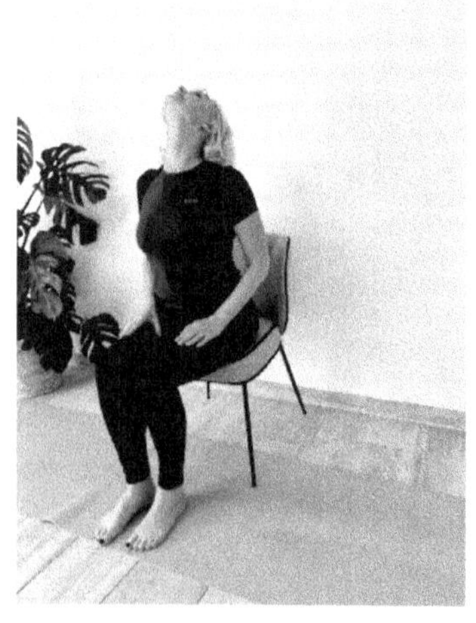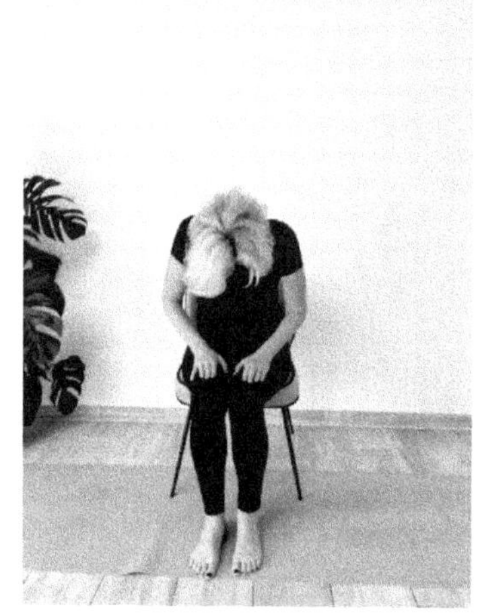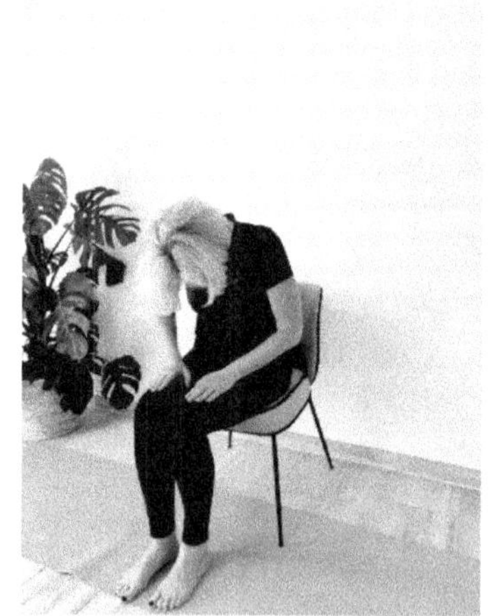

2. **Seated Twist (Bharadvajasana):** Twisting poses help to increase spinal mobility and improve digestion and elimination. Start by sitting tall in your chair with your feet flat on the floor and your spine erect. Inhale as you lengthen your spine, then exhale as you gently twist to the right, placing your left hand on the outside of your right thigh and your right hand on the back of the chair. Keep both sit bones grounded on the chair and your spine tall as you deepen the twist with each exhale. Hold for a few breaths, then inhale to release and switch sides.

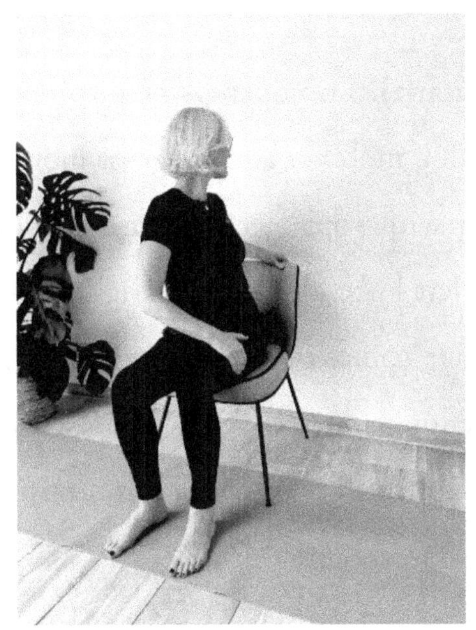 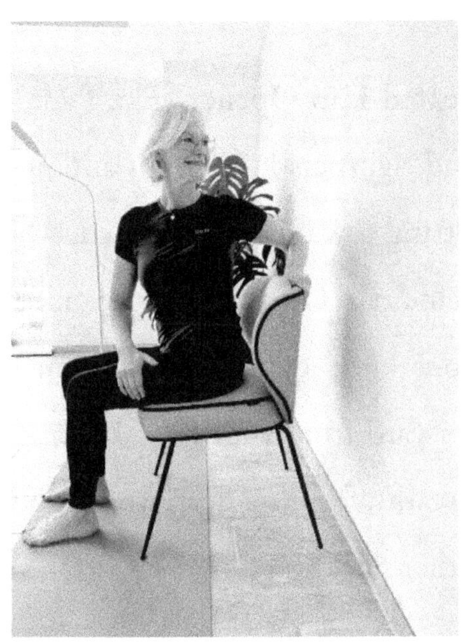

3. **Seated Forward Fold (Paschimottanasana):** Forward folds help to stretch the hamstrings, calves, and lower back, improving flexibility and range of motion in the spine and hips. Start by sitting towards the front edge of your chair with your feet flat on the floor and your spine tall. Inhale as you lengthen your spine, then exhale as you hinge forward from your hips, reaching your hands towards your feet or the floor in front of you. Keep your spine long and your chest open as you fold forward, feeling a gentle stretch along the back of your legs and spine. Hold for a few breaths, then inhale to rise back up to a seated position.

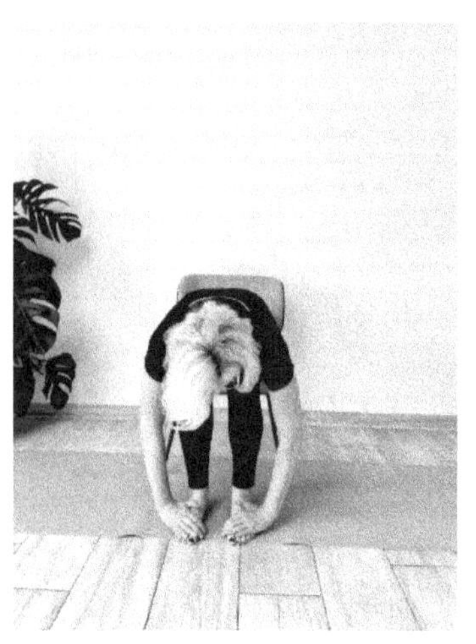
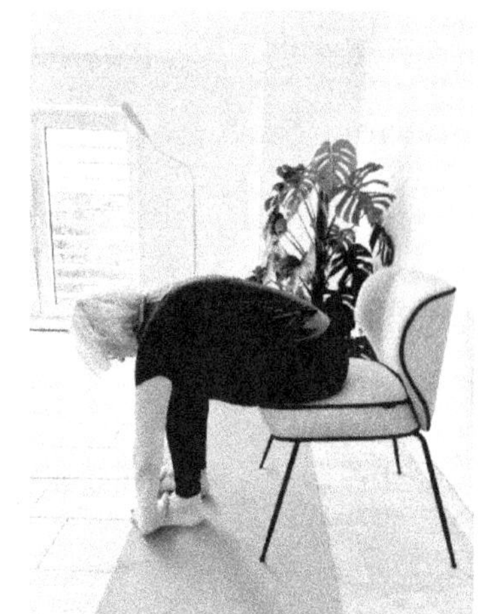
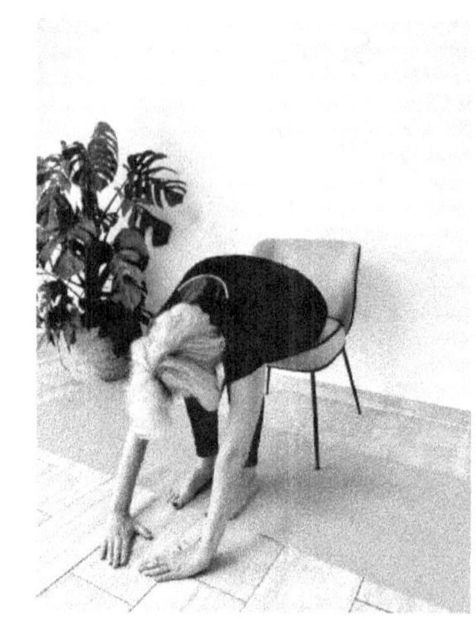

4. **Seated Hip Opener (Eka Pada Rajakapotasana):** Hip openers help to release tension and tightness in the hips and pelvis, improving mobility and range of motion. Start by sitting towards the front edge of your chair with your feet flat on the floor and your spine tall. Cross your right ankle over your left knee, flexing your right foot to protect your knee joint. Inhale as you lengthen your spine, then exhale as you gently hinge forward from your hips, keeping your spine long and your chest open. Hold for a few breaths, feeling a deep stretch in the outer hip and glute of your right leg. Repeat on the other side.

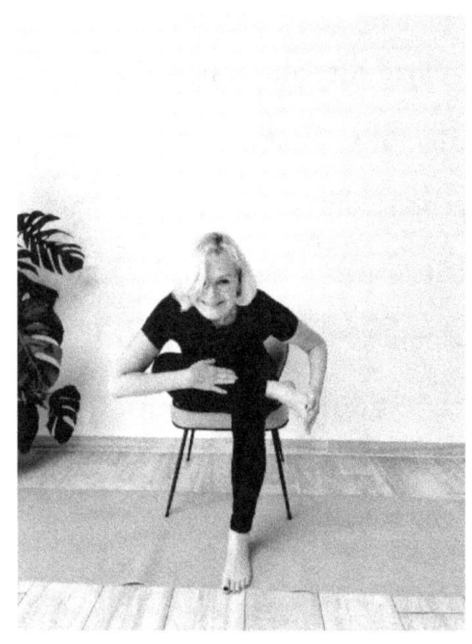
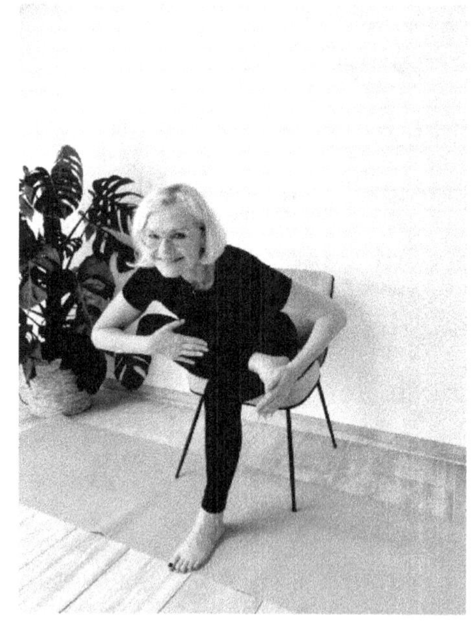

5. **Seated Shoulder Opener:** Shoulder openers help to release tension and tightness in the shoulders and upper back, improving mobility and range of motion. Start by sitting tall in your chair with your feet flat on the floor and your spine erect. Interlace your fingers behind your back, squeezing your shoulder blades together and opening your chest. Inhale as you lift your arms away from your body, feeling a stretch across the front of your chest and shoulders. Hold for a few breaths, then exhale to release and repeat as needed.

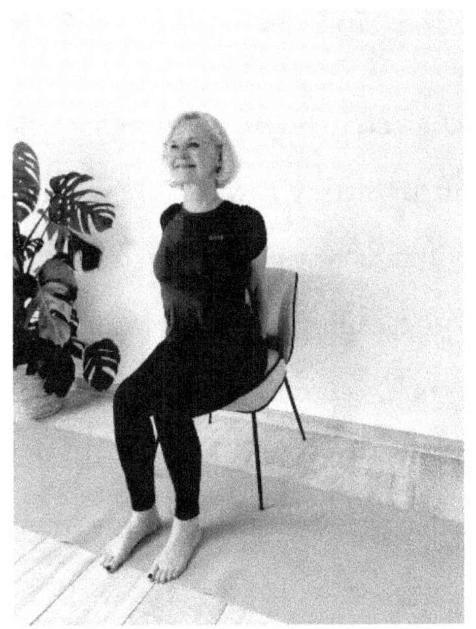 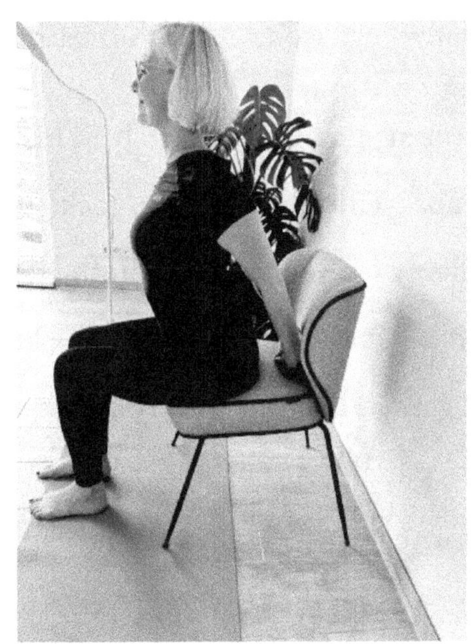

Day 3 – Day 10 – Day 17 – Day 24: Poses for Heart Health

Maintaining heart health is crucial for overall well-being and vitality. Chair Yoga offers a variety of poses and exercises that can help improve circulation, reduce stress, and support heart health. In this section, we'll explore some specific poses and techniques to promote cardiovascular health and strengthen the heart.

Start your daily Yoga Routines with Breathwork and Warm-Up Exercises.

1. **Seated Cat-Cow Stretch:** This classic yoga stretch helps to mobilize the spine and improve flexibility in the back and torso. Start by sitting towards the front edge of your chair with your feet flat on the floor and your hands resting on your knees. Inhale as you arch your back and lift your chest towards the ceiling, drawing your shoulder blades together. Exhale as you round your spine and tuck your chin towards your chest, feeling a stretch along your upper back. Continue to move through this seated cat-cow stretch, flowing with your breath and exploring the full range of motion in your spine.

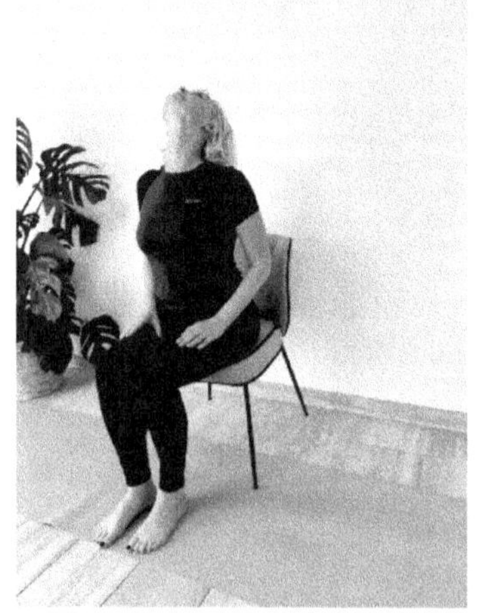 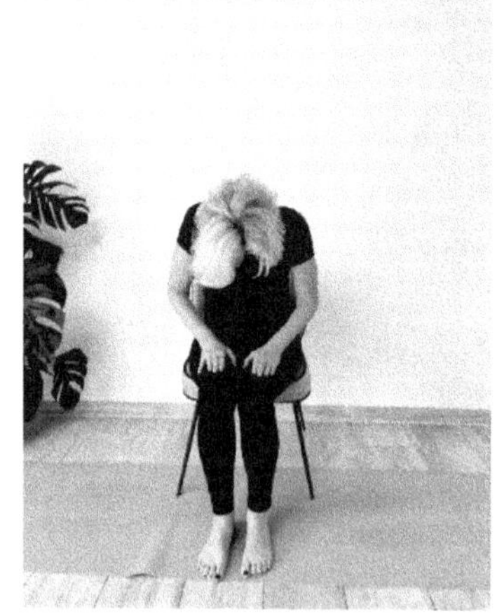 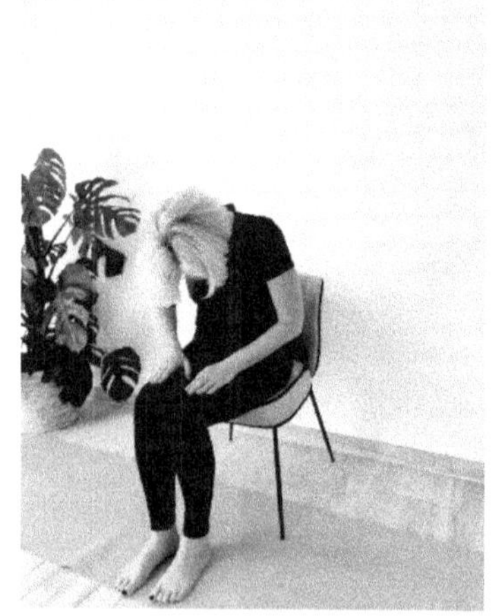

2. **Seated Twist (Bharadvajasana):** Twisting poses help to increase spinal mobility and improve digestion and elimination. Start by sitting tall in your chair with your feet flat on the floor and your spine erect. Inhale as you lengthen your spine, then exhale as you gently twist to the right, placing your left hand on the outside of your right thigh and your right hand on the back of the chair. Keep both sit bones grounded on the chair and your spine tall as you deepen the twist with each exhale. Hold for a few breaths, then inhale to release and switch sides.

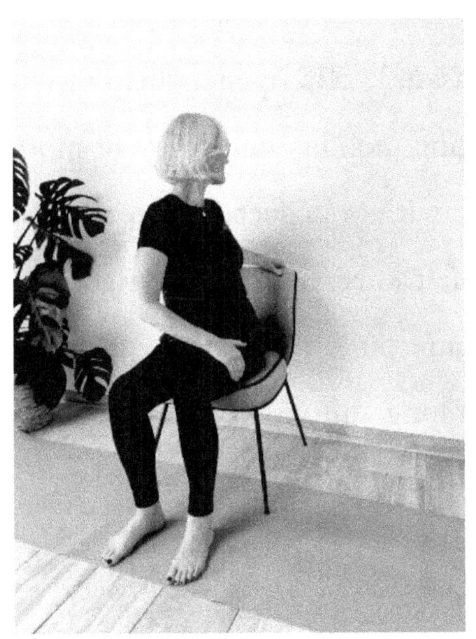 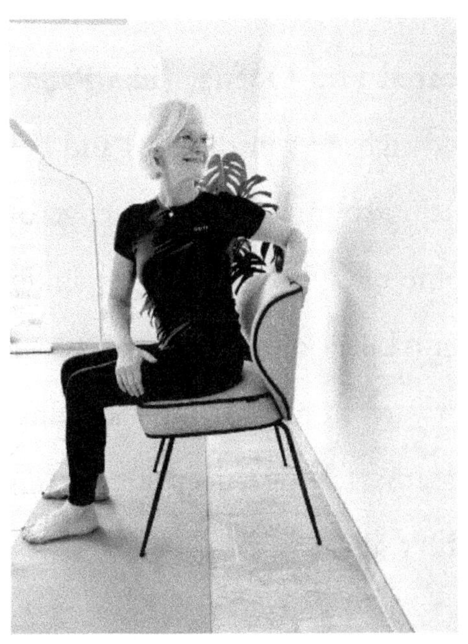

3. **Seated Forward Fold (Paschimottanasana):** Forward folds help to stretch the hamstrings, calves, and lower back, improving flexibility and range of motion in the spine and hips. Start by sitting towards the front edge of your chair with your feet flat on the floor and your spine tall. Inhale as you lengthen your spine, then exhale as you hinge forward from your hips, reaching your hands towards your feet or the floor in front of you. Keep your spine long and your chest open as you fold forward, feeling a gentle stretch along the back of your legs and spine. Hold for a few breaths, then inhale to rise back up to a seated position.

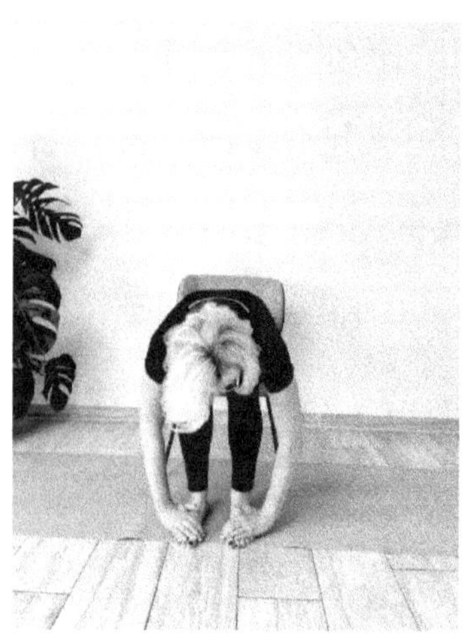 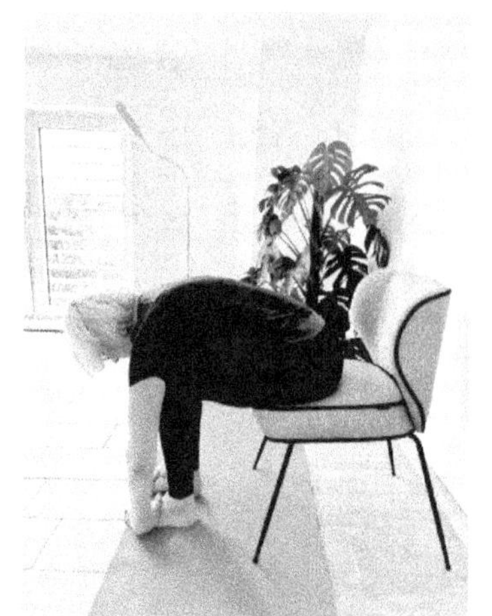 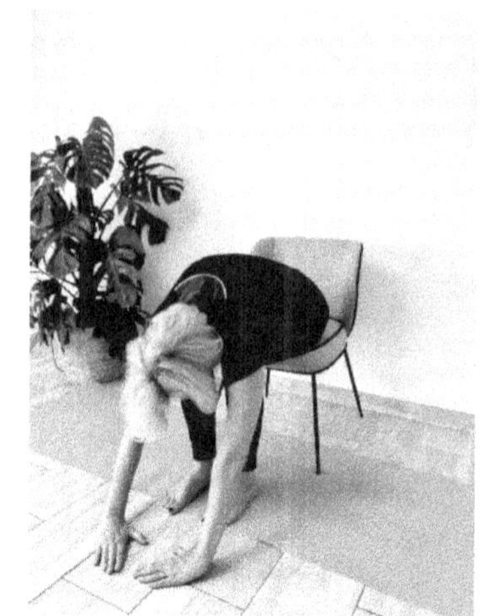

4. **Seated Hip Opener (Eka Pada Rajakapotasana):** Hip openers help to release tension and tightness in the hips and pelvis, improving mobility and range of motion. Start by sitting towards the front edge of your chair with your feet flat on the floor and your spine tall. Cross your right ankle over your left knee, flexing your right foot to protect your knee joint. Inhale as you lengthen your spine, then exhale as you gently hinge forward from your hips, keeping your spine long and your chest open. Hold for a few breaths, feeling a deep stretch in the outer hip and glute of your right leg. Repeat on the other side.

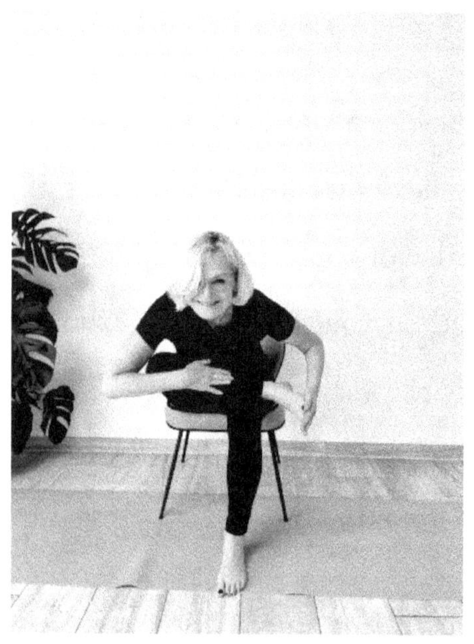 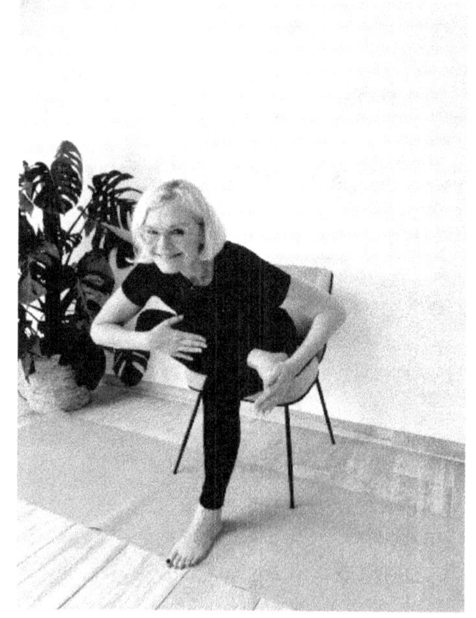

5. **Seated Shoulder Opener:** Shoulder openers help to release tension and tightness in the shoulders and upper back, improving mobility and range of motion. Start by sitting tall in your chair with your feet flat on the floor and your spine erect. Interlace your fingers behind your back, squeezing your shoulder blades together and opening your chest. Inhale as you lift your arms away from your body, feeling a stretch across the front of your chest and shoulders. Hold for a few breaths, then exhale to release and repeat as needed.

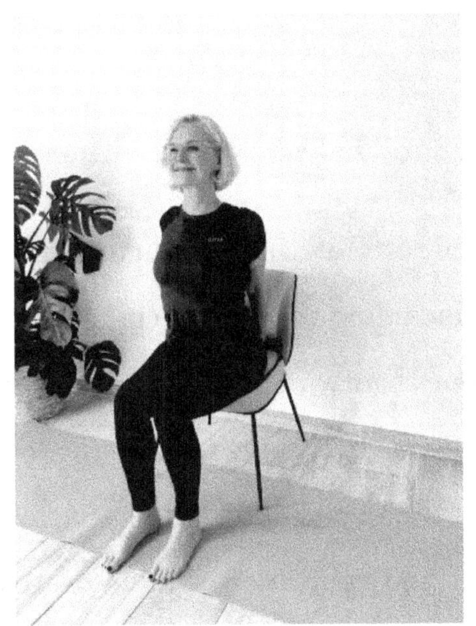
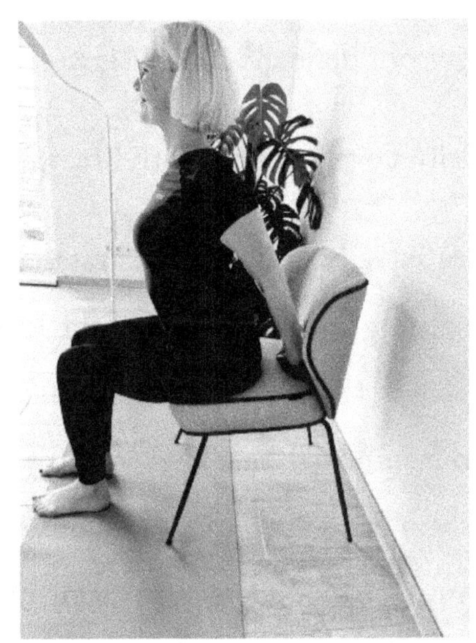

Day 4 – Day 11 – Day 18 – Day 25: Building Strength

Strength is the foundation of mobility and stability, providing support for everyday activities and promoting overall well-being. Chair Yoga offers a gentle yet effective approach to building strength, allowing you to strengthen key muscle groups without putting undue strain on your joints. In this section, we'll explore some simple yet powerful exercises to help you build strength and feel more confident and capable in your body.

Start your daily Yoga Routines with Breathwork and Warm-Up Exercises.

1. **Seated Chair Pose (Utkatasana):** Chair pose is a dynamic strength-building exercise that targets the muscles of the lower body, including the quadriceps, glutes, and calves. Start by sitting towards the front edge of your chair with your feet hip-width apart and your spine tall. Inhale as you lift your arms overhead, reaching towards the ceiling. Exhale as you bend your knees and lower your hips towards the floor, as if you were sitting back into a chair. Keep your weight in your heels and your knees stacked over your ankles. Hold for a few breaths, and then inhale to rise back up to a seated position.

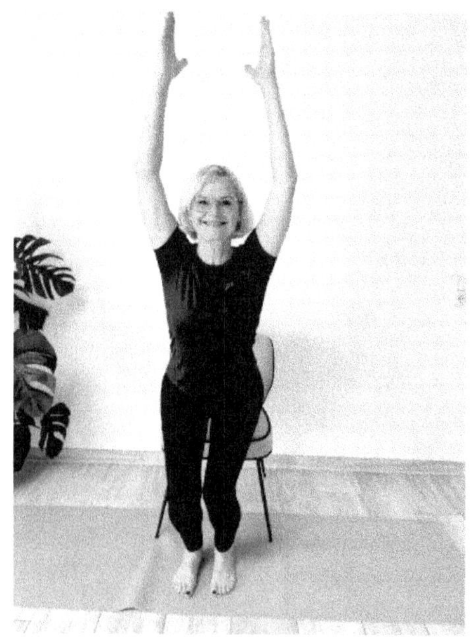
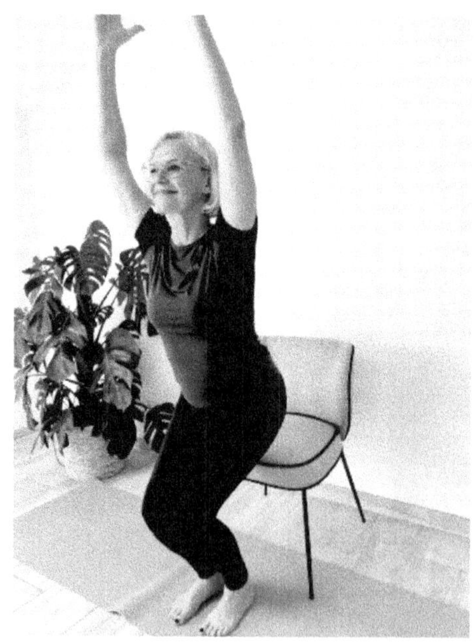

2. **Seated Leg Lifts:** Leg lifts help to strengthen the muscles of the core, hips, and thighs, improving balance and stability. Start by sitting tall in your chair with your feet flat on the floor and your spine erect. Hold onto the sides of the chair for support if needed. Inhale as you extend your right leg out in front of you, lifting it towards hip height. Exhale as you lower your right leg back down to the floor. Repeat on the other side, lifting and lowering your left leg. Continue to alternate sides, moving with control and engaging your core muscles throughout the movement.

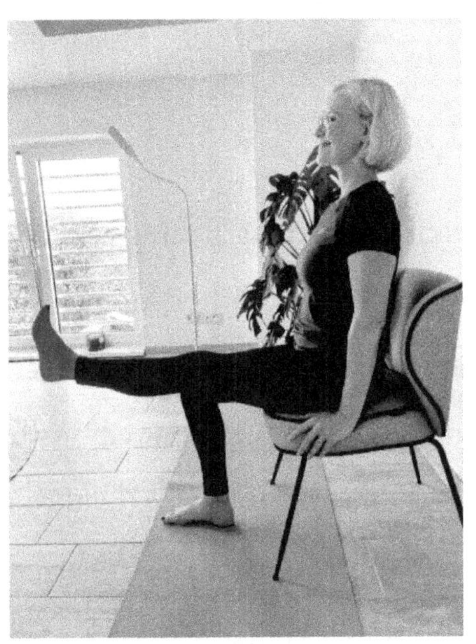 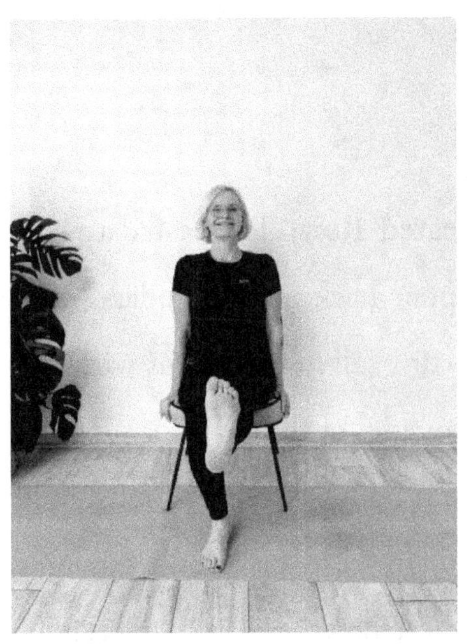

3. **Seated Knee Lifts:** Knee lifts target the muscles of the core and hip flexors, helping to improve posture and stability. Start by sitting tall in your chair with your feet flat on the floor and your spine erect. Inhale as you lift your right knee towards your chest, bringing it as close to your body as comfortably possible. Exhale as you lower your right foot back down to the floor. Repeat on the other side, lifting and lowering your left knee. Continue to alternate sides, moving with control and focusing on engaging your core muscles.

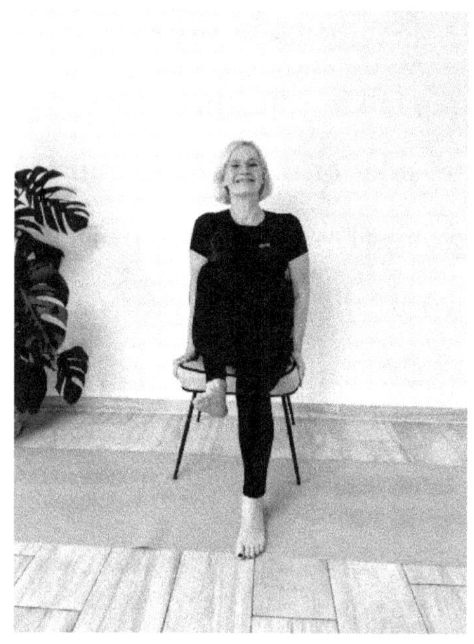 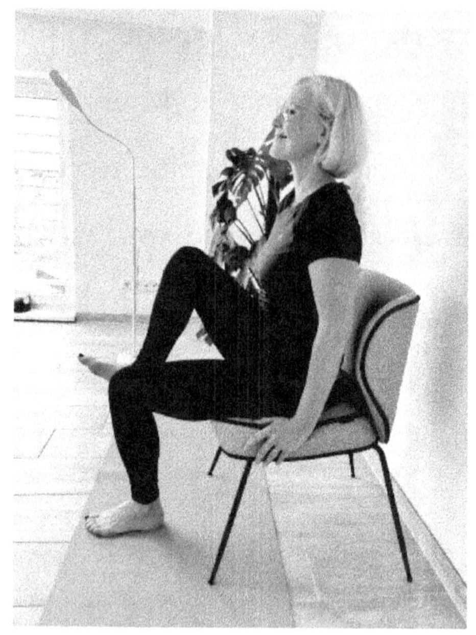

4.   **Seated Row:** The seated row is a great exercise for strengthening the muscles of the upper back and shoulders, helping to improve posture and reduce tension. Start by sitting tall in your chair with your feet flat on the floor and your spine erect. Hold onto the sides of the chair for support if needed. Inhale as you draw your elbows back towards your body, squeezing your shoulder blades together. Exhale as you extend your arms back out in front of you, lengthening through your spine. Repeat this movement, drawing your elbows back and squeezing your shoulder blades together with each repetition.

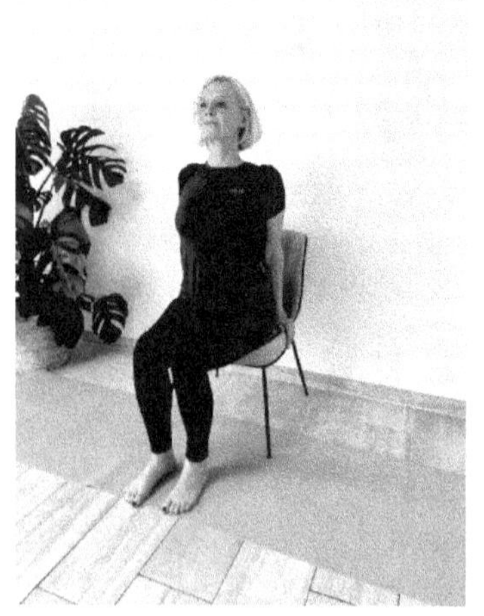 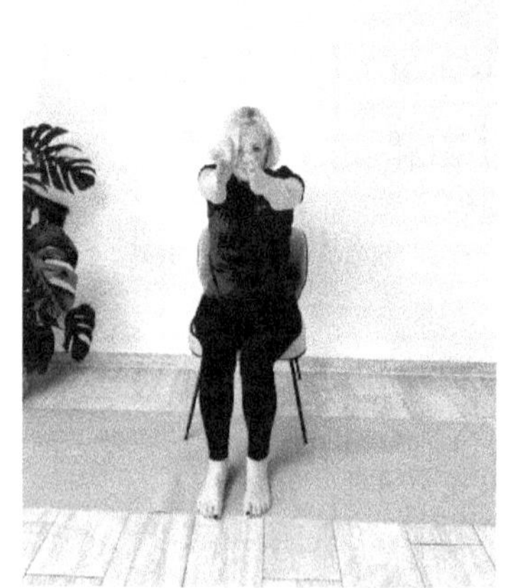 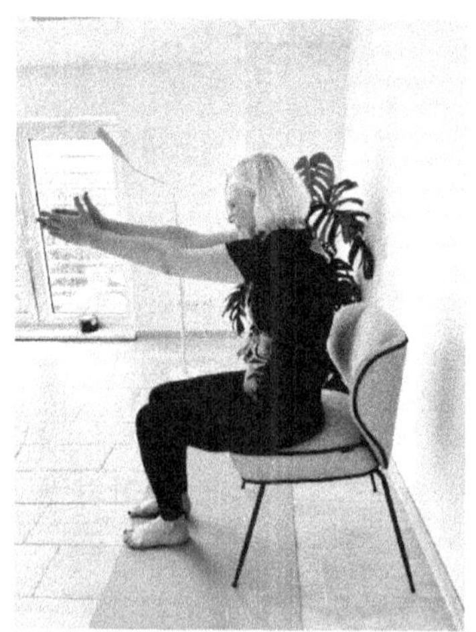

5. **Seated Bicep Curls:** Bicep curls target the muscles of the arms, helping to improve strength and tone in the biceps and forearms. Start by sitting tall in your chair with your feet flat on the floor and your spine erect. Hold onto a pair of light hand weights or water bottles in each hand, palms facing up. Inhale as you bend your elbows and curl the weights towards your shoulders, keeping your elbows close to your body. Exhale as you lower the weights back down to your sides. Repeat this movement, curling the weights towards your shoulders with each repetition.

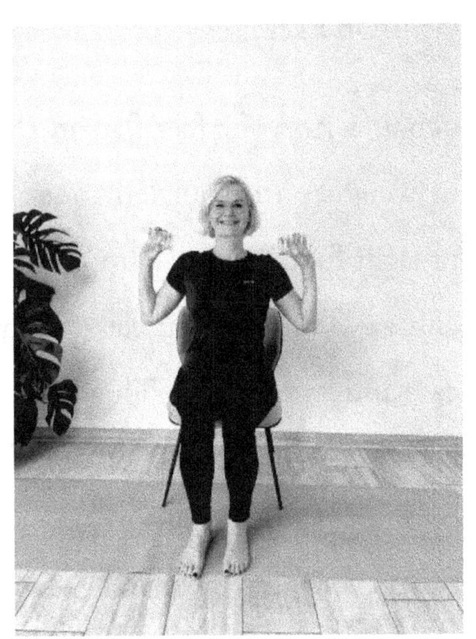 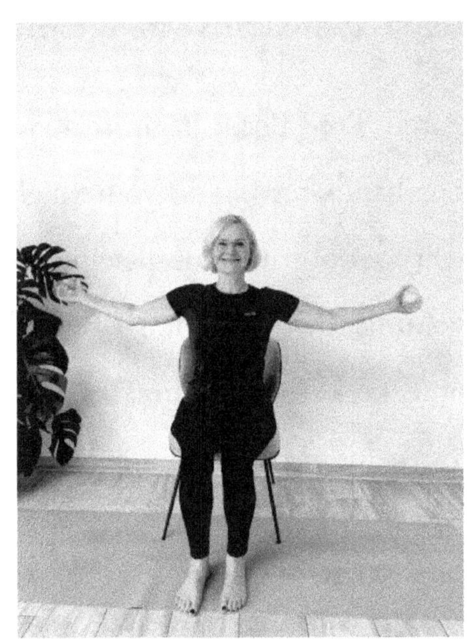

Day 5 – Day 12 – Day 19 – Day 26: Balance Enhancement

As we embark on our Chair Yoga journey, it's important to lay a strong foundation, starting with balance enhancement. These five exercises are tailored for adult beginners, and designed to improve stability, cultivate body awareness, and lay the groundwork for a fulfilling Chair Yoga practice.

Start your daily Yoga Routines with Breathwork and Warm-Up Exercises.

1. **Seated Tree Pose:** Begin seated tall in your chair with your feet flat on the floor and your hands resting on your thighs. Shift your weight onto your left foot and lift your right foot off the floor, placing the sole of your right foot on your left inner thigh or calf, avoiding the knee. Find your balance and engage your core muscles to stabilize your spine. Hold for a few breaths, then gently release and switch sides. This variation of Tree Pose helps improve balance and focus while seated.

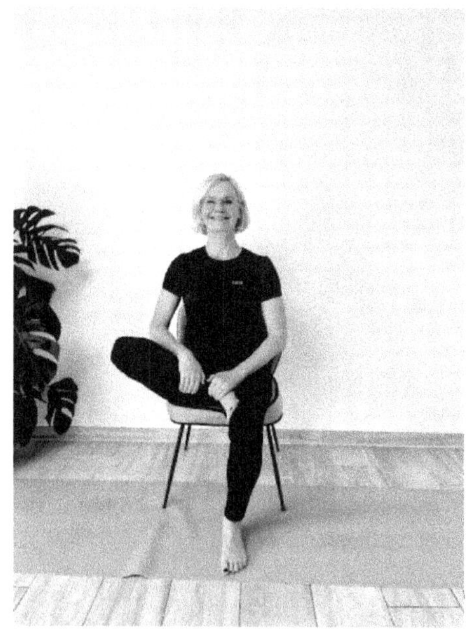
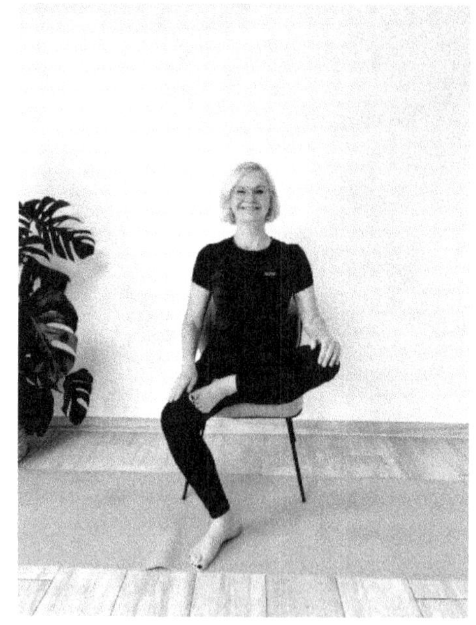

2. **Seated Side Leg Lifts:** Sit towards the front edge of your chair with your feet flat on the floor and your hands resting on your thighs. Inhale deeply, and then exhale as you lift your right leg out to the side, keeping it straight and parallel to the floor. Engage your core muscles to support your spine and maintain stability. Hold for a few breaths, and then lower your leg back down. Repeat on the left side. Seated side leg lifts strengthen the muscles of the hips and thighs, improving stability and mobility.

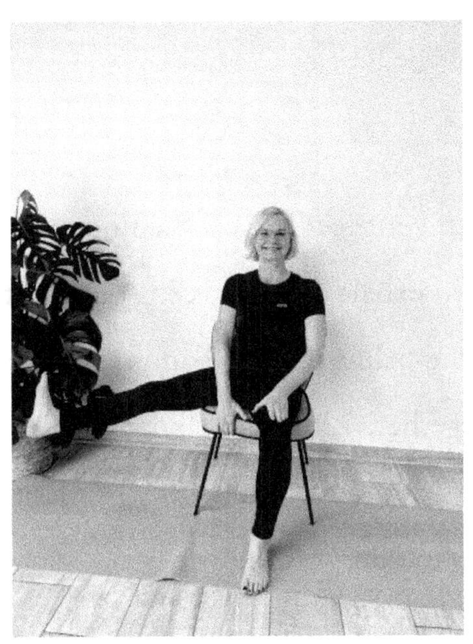 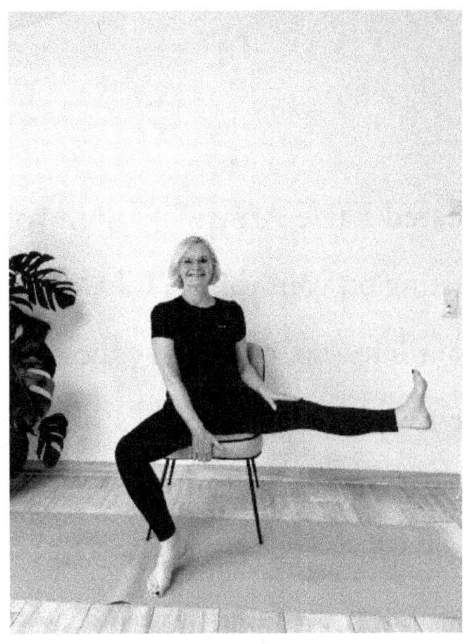

3. **Seated Warrior III:** Sit tall in your chair with your feet flat on the floor and your hands resting on your thighs. Inhale deeply, then exhale as you hinge forward from your hips, extending your right leg back behind you and reaching your arms forward, parallel to the floor. Keep your spine long and your chest open, and engage your core muscles to stabilize your body. Hold for a few breaths, then return to an upright position and switch sides. Seated Warrior III strengthens the muscles of the legs, core, and back, improving balance and posture.

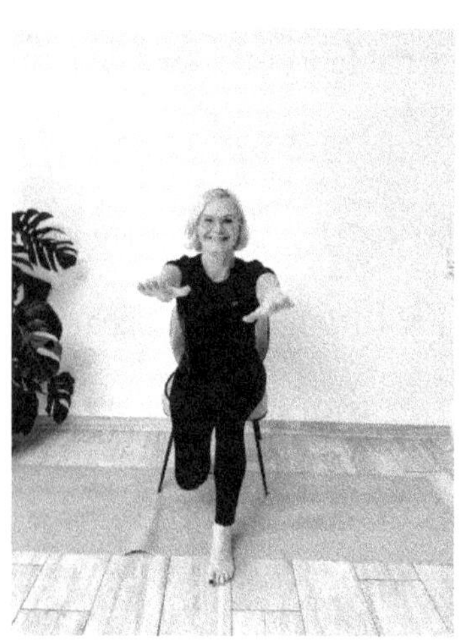
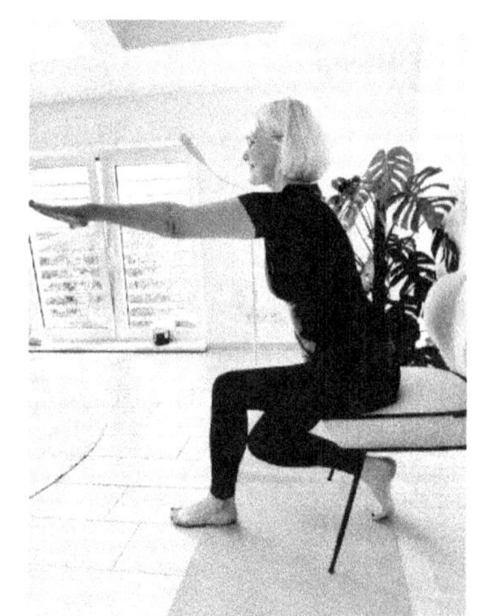
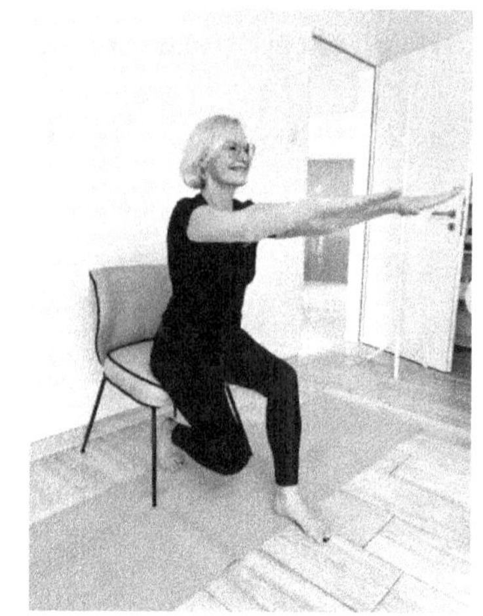

4. **Seated Eagle Arms:** Sit tall in your chair with your feet flat on the floor and your hands resting on your thighs. Inhale deeply, and then exhale as you sweep your right arm under your left arm, crossing at the elbows. Bring the palms of your hands together if possible, or simply press the backs of your hands together. Lift your elbows slightly and feel a stretch across your upper back and shoulders. Hold for a few breaths, then release and switch sides. Seated Eagle Arms stretch the shoulders and upper back, releasing tension and improving posture.

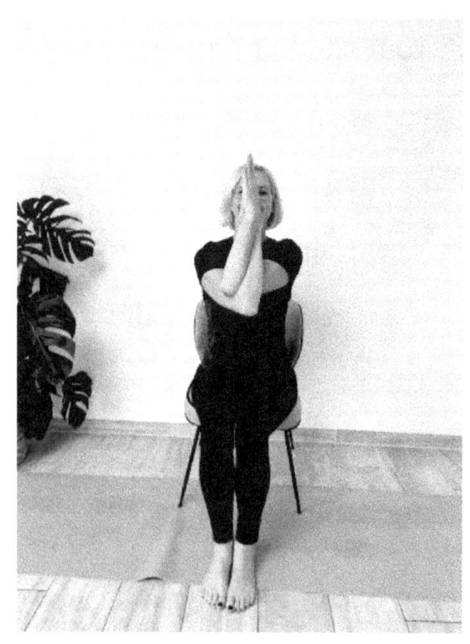
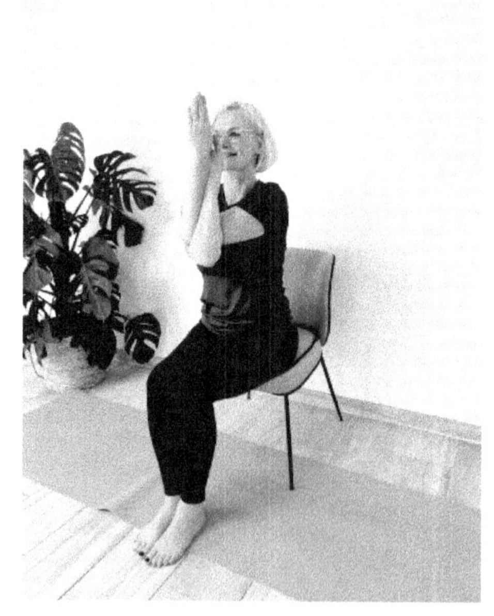

5. **Seated Knee Raises:** Sit tall in your chair with your feet flat on the floor. Inhale deeply, and then exhale as you lift your right knee towards your chest, bringing it as close as comfortably possible. Hold for a few breaths, and then lower your foot back down to the floor. Repeat on the left side. Focus on engaging your core and maintaining stability through your standing leg. This exercise strengthens the muscles of the hip and thigh while improving balance and coordination.

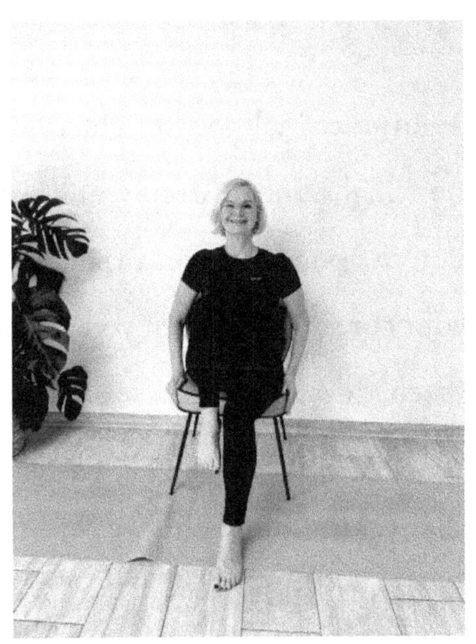 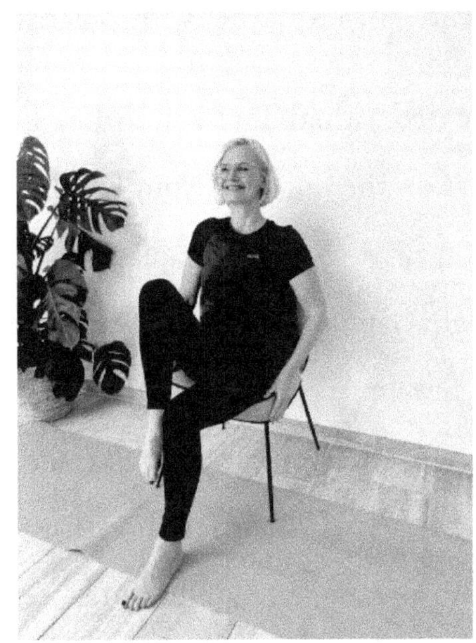

Day 6 – Day 13 – Day 20 – Day 27: Mobility and Strength

As we embark on our Chair Yoga journey, let's explore five beginner-friendly exercises to enhance mobility and build strength in key areas of the body.

Start your daily Yoga Routines with Breathwork and Warm-Up Exercises.

1. **Seated Spinal Twist with Leg Extension:** Begin seated tall in your chair with your feet flat on the floor and your hands resting on your thighs. Inhale deeply, and then exhale as you twist to the right, placing your left hand on the outside of your right knee and your right hand on the back of the chair. Engage your core and lengthen your spine. Hold for a few breaths, then return to center and switch sides. To add a leg extension, inhale deeply, then exhale as you extend your right leg out in front of you while twisting to the right. Hold for a few breaths, then return to center and switch sides. This exercise improves spinal mobility and strengthens the core and legs.

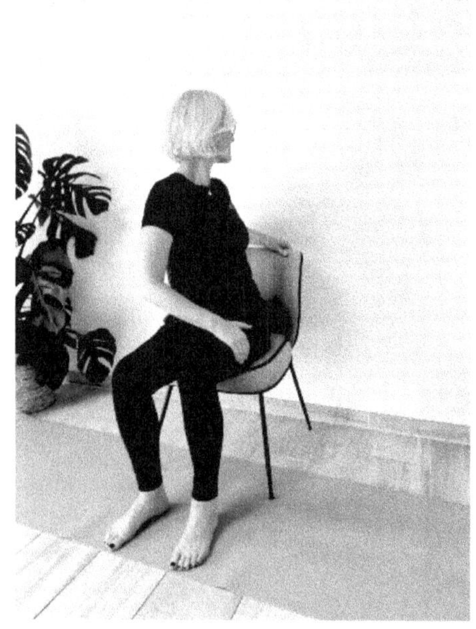
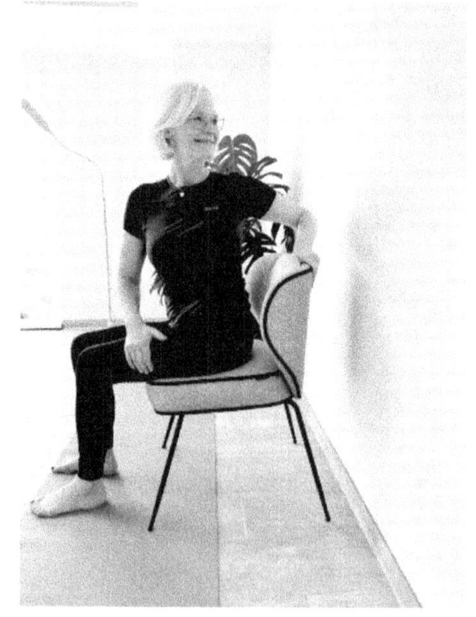

2. **Seated Squats:** Sit towards the front edge of your chair with your feet flat on the floor and your knees aligned with your ankles. Inhale deeply, then exhale as you engage your core and lower your hips towards the floor, as if you're sitting back into an imaginary chair. Keep your weight in your heels and your knees aligned with your ankles. Inhale to return to the starting position. Repeat for several repetitions, focusing on controlled movements and engaging the muscles of the legs and glutes. Seated squats strengthen the muscles of the lower body, improving mobility and stability.

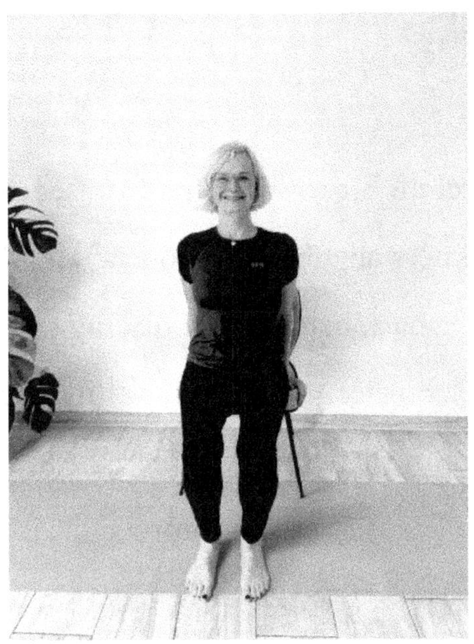

3. **Seated Warrior II:** Sit tall in your chair with your feet flat on the floor and your hands resting on your thighs. Inhale deeply, and then exhale as you extend your right leg out to the side, keeping it straight and parallel to the floor. Turn your torso to the right, reaching your right arm forward and your left arm back, palms facing down. Engage your core and lengthen your spine. Hold for a few breaths, then return to center and switch sides. Seated Warrior II strengthens the muscles of the legs, hips, and core, improving mobility and stability.

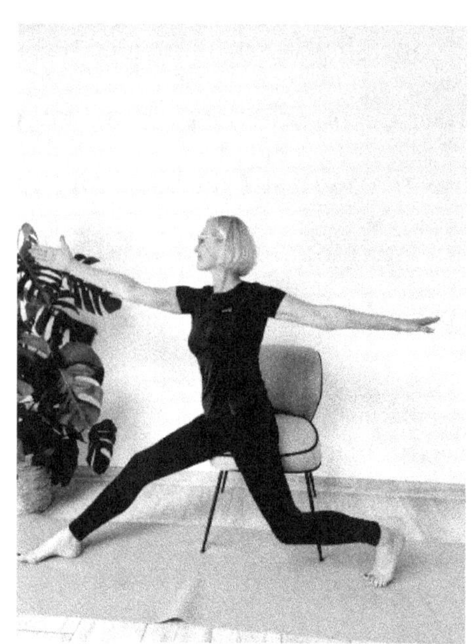 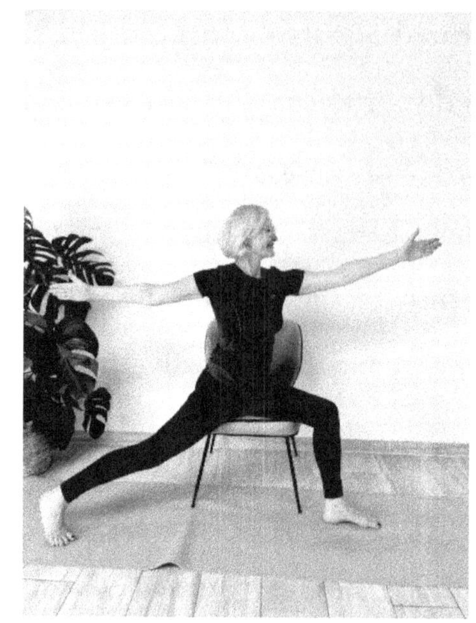

4. **Seated Hip Flexor Stretch:** Sit towards the front edge of your chair with your feet flat on the floor and your knees aligned with your ankles. Inhale deeply, and then exhale as you extend your right leg back behind you, placing the top of your foot on the floor and bending your left knee. Engage your core and lift your torso upright. Hold for a few breaths, feeling a stretch in the front of your right hip and thigh. Return to center and switch sides. Seated hip flexor stretches improve flexibility and mobility in the hips and thighs.

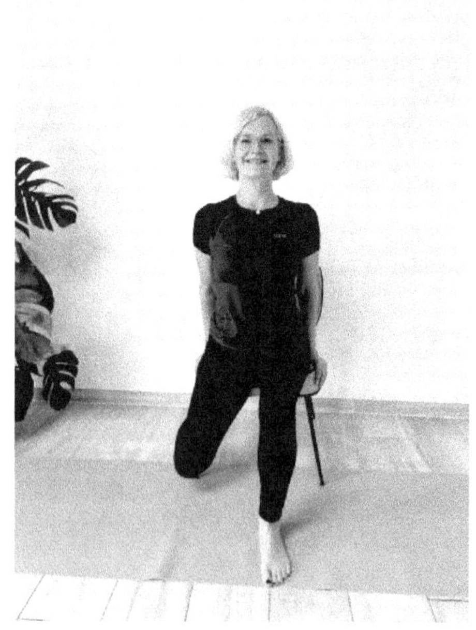 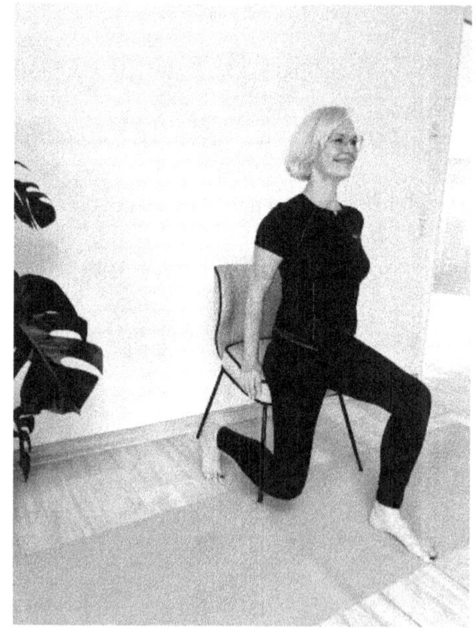

5. **Seated Cat-Cow Stretch:** Sit tall in your chair with your feet flat on the floor and your hands resting on your thighs. Inhale deeply, and then exhale as you round your spine, tucking your chin towards your chest and drawing your navel towards your spine. Inhale as you arch your back, lifting your chest towards the ceiling and drawing your shoulder blades together. Continue to flow between these two movements with your breath, moving slowly and mindfully. Seated cat-cow stretches improve spinal mobility and release tension in the back and neck.

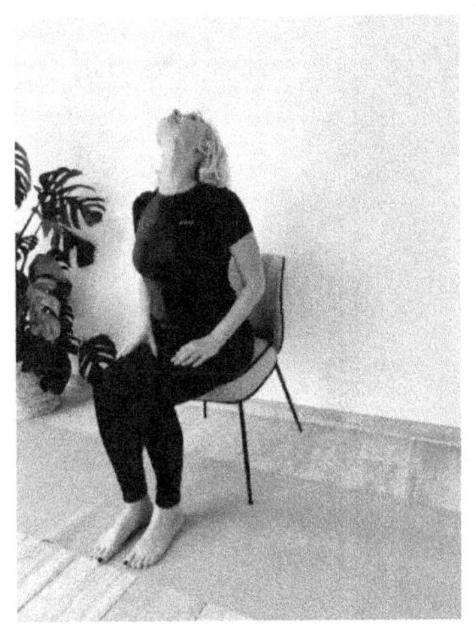
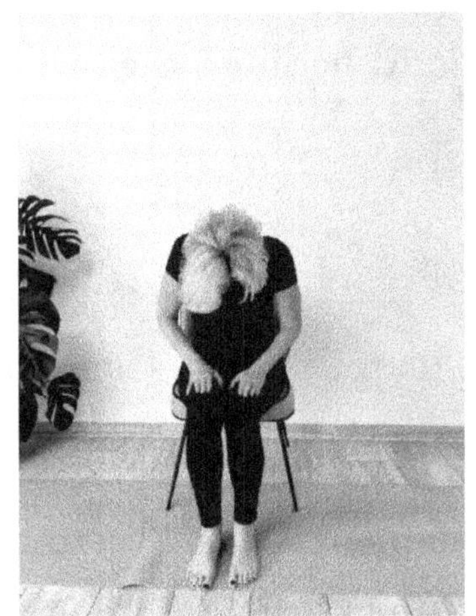
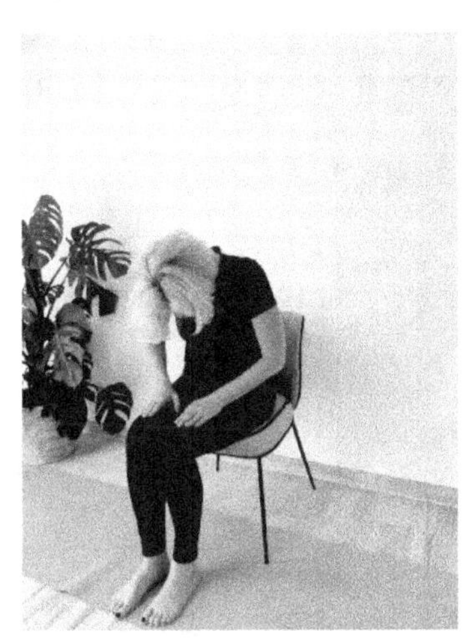

Day 7 – Day 14 – Day 21 – Day 28: Relaxation and Meditation

As we embark on this journey of relaxation and meditation, let's take a moment to breathe deeply and settle into our chairs. In today's fast-paced world, it's all too easy to get caught up in the hustle and bustle of everyday life. With gentle movements and mindful breathwork, we can create a sense of peace and calm within ourselves, no matter what challenges life throws our way. Together, we'll cultivate a sense of ease, balance, and inner harmony that will stay with us long after we roll up our yoga mats. Let's begin!

1. **Seated Breath Awareness:** Begin by sitting tall in your chair with your feet flat on the floor and yourhands resting on your thighs. Close your eyes if comfortable or soften your gaze. Take a few deep breaths, inhaling through your nose and exhaling through your mouth. As you breathe, bring your awareness to the sensations of your breath moving in and out of your body. Notice the rise and fall of your chest and belly with each inhale and exhale. Allow your breath to become slow, smooth, and steady. Spend a few moments simply observing your breath, without trying to change it in any way. This practice of breath awareness helps to calm the mind and anchor you in the present moment.

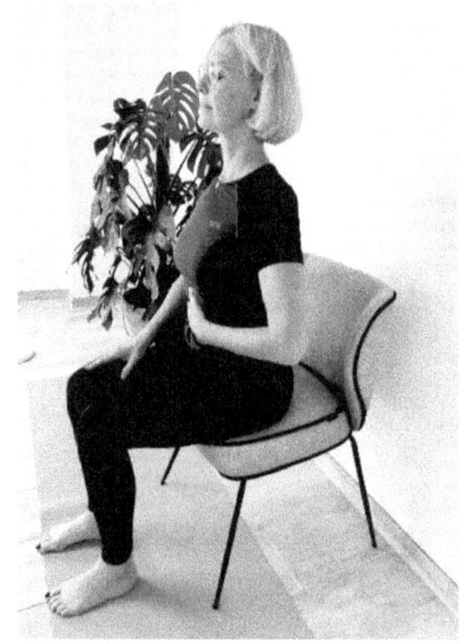

2. **Seated Shoulder and Neck Release:** Sit tall in your chair with your feet flat on the floor and your hands resting on your thighs. Inhale deeply, then exhale as you drop your right ear towards your right shoulder, stretching the left side of your neck. Hold for a few breaths, then return to center and repeat on the left side. Next, inhale deeply and shrug your shoulders up towards your ears, then exhale and release them down, feeling the tension melt away. Repeat this shoulder roll a few times, allowing your shoulders to become heavy and relaxed. This seated shoulder and neck release helps to relieve tension and stress in the upper body.

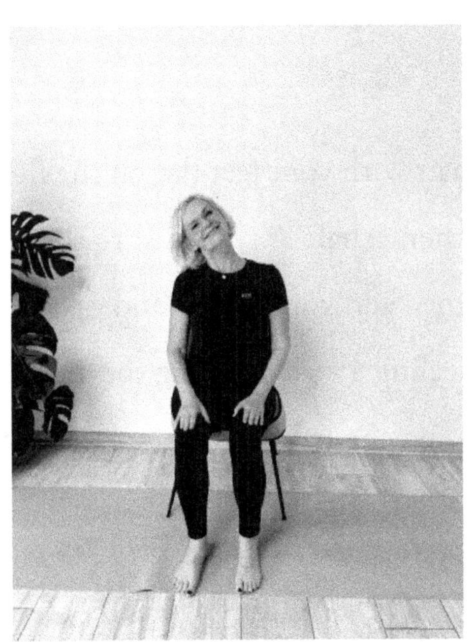 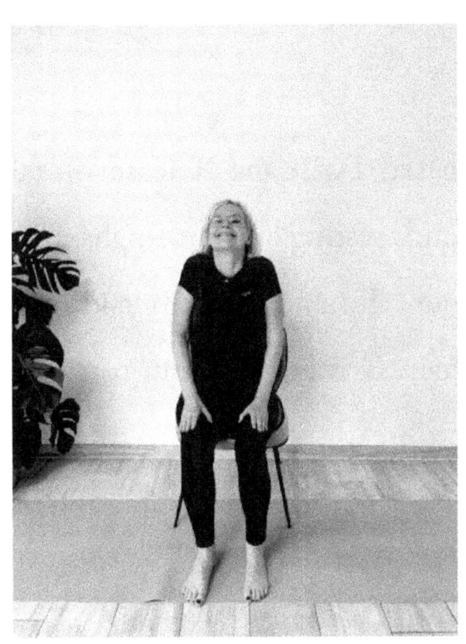

3. **Seated Relaxation Pose:** Sit comfortably in your chair with your feet flat on the floor and your hands resting on your thighs. Close your eyes if comfortable, or soften your gaze. Take a few deep breaths to settle into the present moment. Allow your body to relax completely, from the crown of your head to the tips of your toes. Release any tension or tightness you may be holding onto, and surrender to the support of the chair beneath you. Imagine each inhale bringing a sense of calm and relaxation into your body, and each exhale releasing any remaining tension or stress. Rest in this seated relaxation pose for a few minutes, allowing yourself to fully unwind and let go.

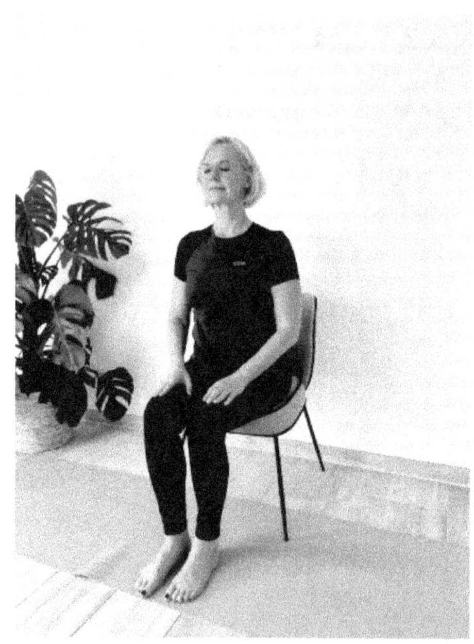

4.   **Seated Twist and Release:** Sit tall in your chair with your feet flat on the floor and your hands resting on your thighs. Inhale deeply, then exhale as you twist to the right, placing your left hand on the outside of your right knee and your right hand on the back of the chair. Gently twist your torso to the right, feeling a stretch along the spine. Hold for a few breaths, then return to center and repeat on the left side. This seated twist helps to release tension in the spine and improve spinal mobility.

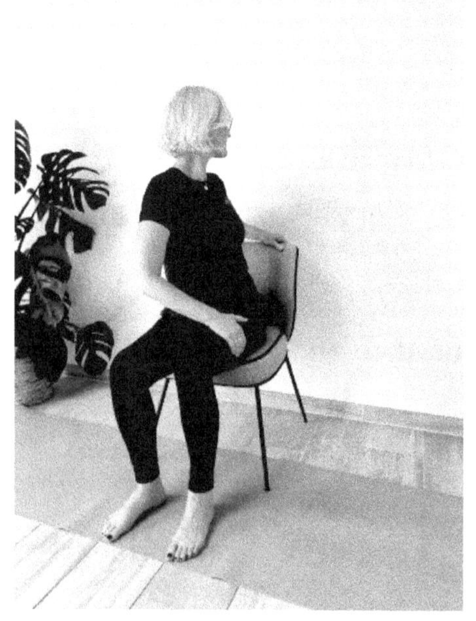

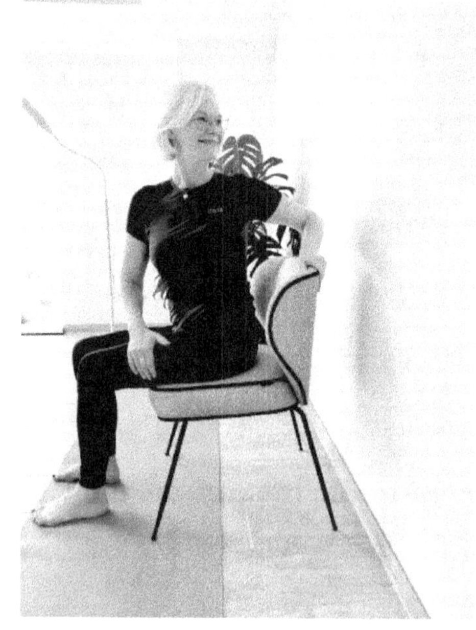

5. **Seated Mindful Eating:** Sit comfortably in your chair with a small snack or piece of fruit in front of you. Take a moment to observe the snack with all your senses. Notice its color, texture, and smell. Take a few deep breaths to center yourself, then pick up the snack and bring it to your mouth. Take a small bite and chew slowly, paying attention to the taste and texture of the food. Notice the sensations of chewing and swallowing. Continue to eat mindfully, savoring each bite and fully experiencing the act of eating. This practice of mindful eating can help to promote relaxation and cultivate a sense of gratitude for the nourishment your body receives.

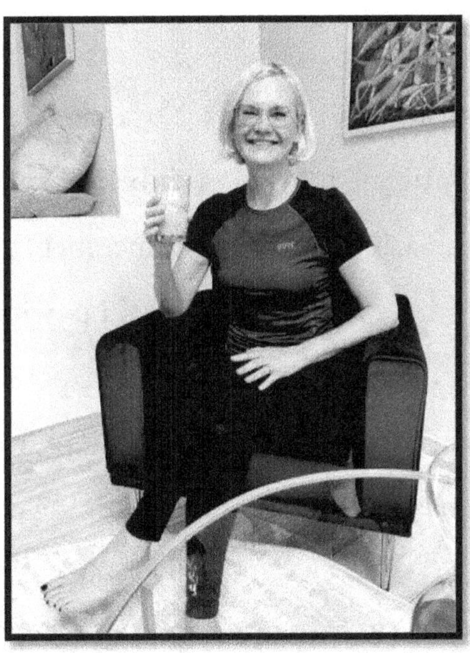

Wishing you continued joy and success on your Chair Yoga journey!

We'll see you in the next level! Keep up the fantastic work!

PART 5

Level-Up with Chair Yoga for Intermediate

Congratulations on completing the 28-day Chair Yoga challenge for beginners! You've shown incredible dedication and commitment to your well-being, and I couldn't be prouder of your accomplishments. Keep up the amazing work, and remember, this is just the beginning of your journey to a healthier, happier life. It's time to level-up with Chair Yoga for intermediate practitioners. In this section, we'll explore more advanced poses and sequences to deepen your practice and take your yoga journey to the next level. We look forward to seeing you continue to thrive as you explore the next levels of Chair Yoga. Keep shining bright!

28-Day Chair Yoga Challenge for Intermediate

Dear Chair Yoga Enthusiasts, welcome to the 28-day Chair Yoga challenge for intermediates! I'm thrilled to have you join me as we take our practice to the next level and explore new heights of strength, flexibility, and mindfulness. As someone who has dedicated years to practicing and teaching Chair Yoga, I understand the importance of building upon the foundation we've already established.

To kickstart your journey, I've curated seven meticulously detailed exercises that will challenge you to push your boundaries and discover new depths within your practice. These exercises are designed to build upon the skills you've already acquired, helping you refine your movements, deepen your stretches, and cultivate a greater sense of balance and stability.

But the real magic happens with repetition. After completing these initial exercises, I encourage you to continue practicing them diligently for the next three weeks. By repeating these movements, you'll not only become more familiar with them but also refine your technique and deepen your connection to each pose.

Through repetition, you'll find that the movements become smoother, more precise, and more graceful. You'll feel more confident in your practice, knowing that you can move with ease and grace. And most importantly, you'll begin to notice the incredible progress you've made – both physically and mentally.

Remember, the path to success is not always linear. There may be days when you feel challenged or discouraged, but don't let that deter you. Every step you take, every breath you breathe, brings you closer to your goals.

So keep showing up on your mat, keep moving your body with intention, and keep listening to the wisdom of your own body. In the end, you'll emerge stronger, fitter, more mindful, and more serene than ever before. I believe in you, and I'm here to support you every step of the way. Together, let's embrace the journey and celebrate the incredible transformations that lie ahead.

Wishing you continued joy and success on your Chair Yoga journey!

Day 1 – Day 8 – Day 15 – Day 22: Foundation Building Exercises

Today, I'm thrilled to share with you foundation-building exercises specifically designed for intermediate seniors. These exercises will help you deepen your practice, enhance your stability, and strengthen your body from the inside out. Let's dive in!

Start your daily Yoga Routines with Breathwork and Warm-Up Exercises.

1. **Seated Mountain Pose with Arm Variations:** Start by sitting tall in your chair with your feet flat on the floor and your hands resting on your thighs. Inhale deeply as you reach your arms overhead, lengthening your spine and lifting your chest. Exhale as you bring your hands together in prayer position, then inhale and stretch your arms out to the sides, palms facing up. Exhale as you bring your hands back to prayer position. Repeat this sequence several times, moving with your breath. This exercise builds strength in the arms, shoulders, and core while improving posture and stability.

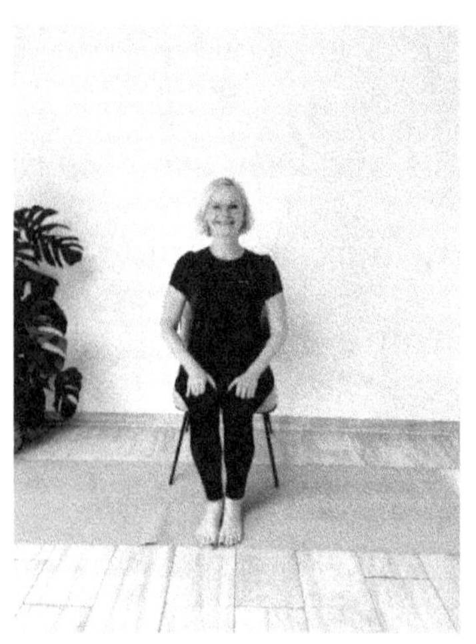
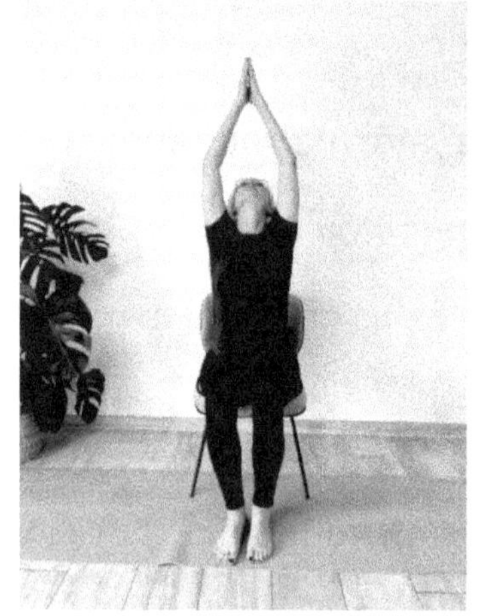
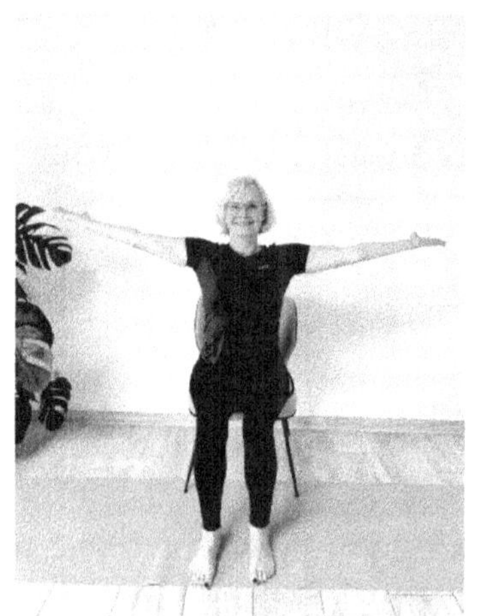

2. **Seated Warrior I:** Sit towards the front edge of your chair with your feet flat on the floor and your hands resting on your thighs. Inhale deeply, then exhale as you extend your right leg back behind you, keeping it straight and strong. Square your hips towards the front of the chair and bend your left knee, bringing it directly over your left ankle. Inhale as you reach your arms overhead, palms facing each other. Hold for a few breaths, then exhale and release. Repeat on the other side. Seated Warrior I strengthens the legs, opens the hips, and improves balance and concentration.

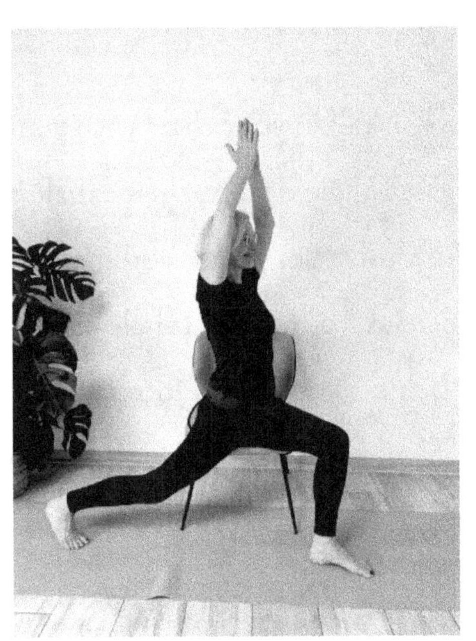 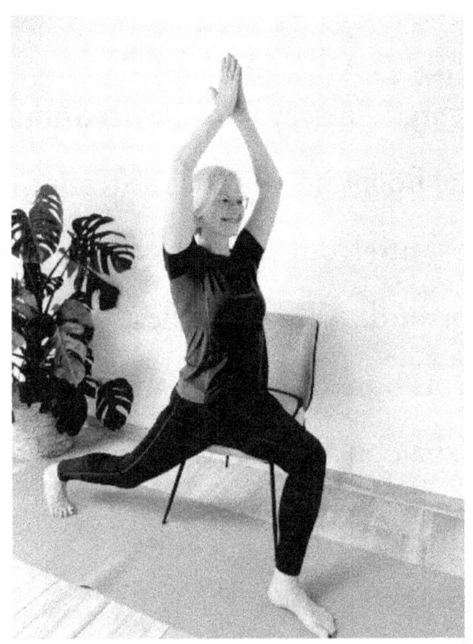

3. **Seated Cat-Cow Stretch:** Begin seated tall in your chair with your feet flat on the floor and your hands resting on your thighs. Inhale deeply as you arch your back, lifting your chest towards the ceiling and drawing your shoulder blades together. Exhale as you round your spine, tucking your chin towards your chest and drawing your navel towards your spine. Continue to flow between these two movements with your breath, moving slowly and mindfully. Seated Cat-Cow Stretch improves spinal mobility and releases tension in the back and neck.

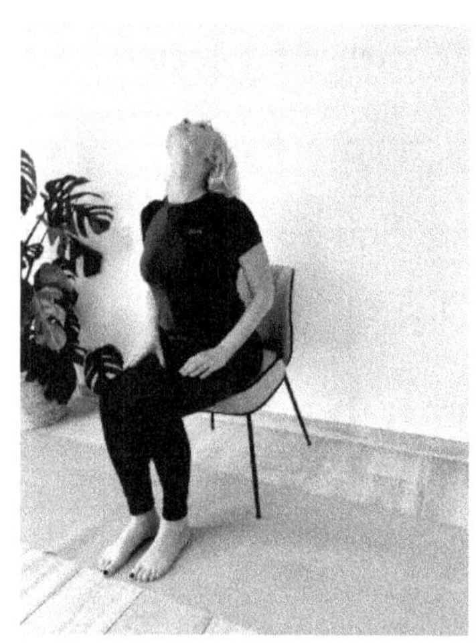 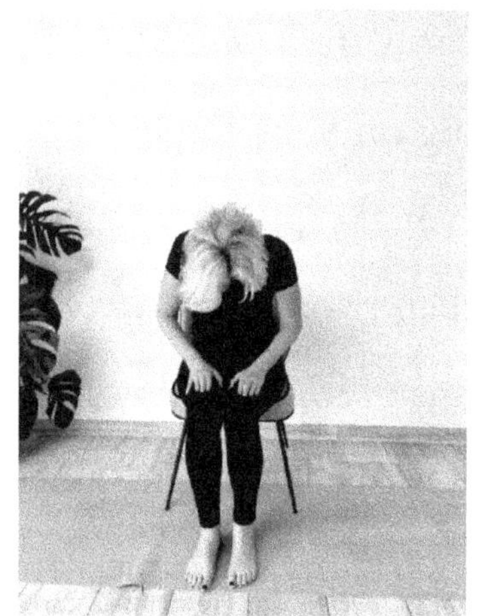 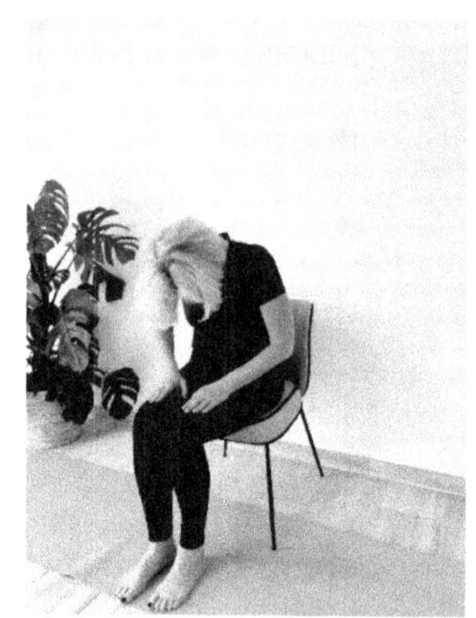

4. **Seated Forward Fold with Shoulder Opener:** Sit tall in your chair with your feet flat on the floor and your hands resting on your thighs. Inhale deeply, then exhale as you hinge forward from your hips, bringing your chest towards your thighs and reaching your arms forward. Allow your head to hang heavy and relax your neck. Inhale as you reach your arms out to the sides and bring your hands behind your back, interlacing your fingers. Exhale as you gently lift your hands away from your body, opening your chest and shoulders. Hold for a few breaths, then release and return to an upright position. Seated Forward Fold with Shoulder Opener stretches the hamstrings, releases tension in the shoulders, and improves spinal flexibility.

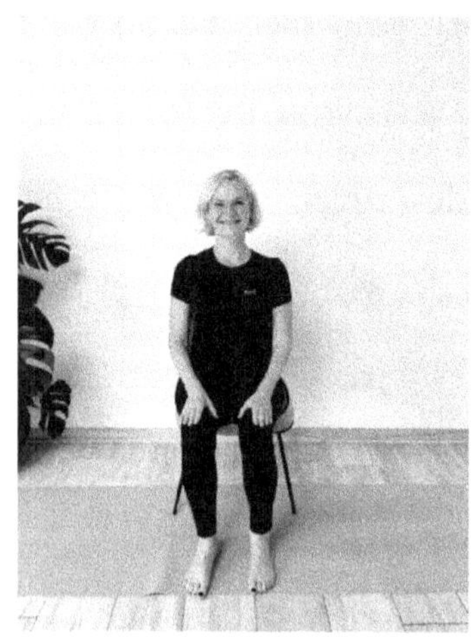 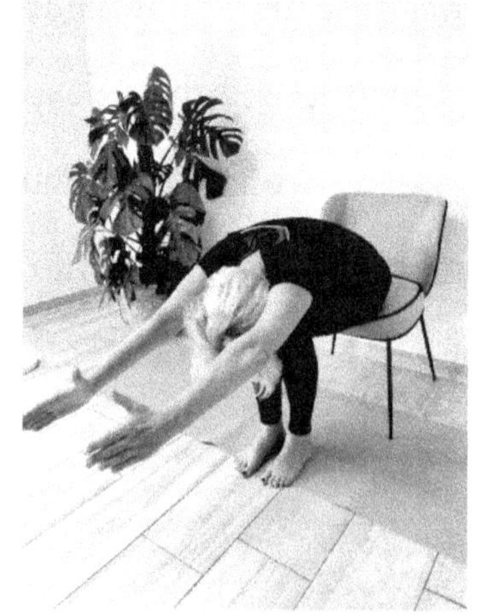 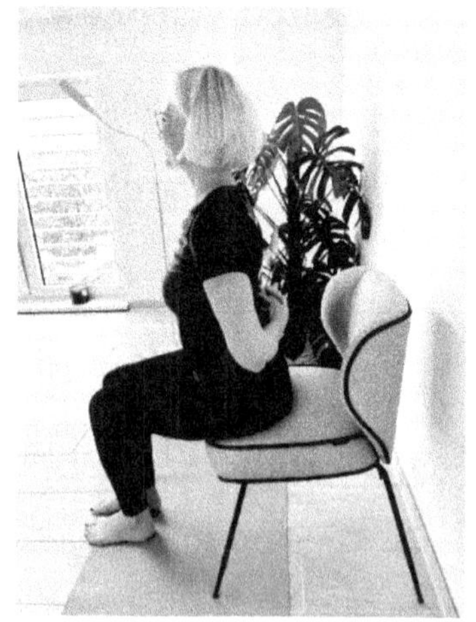

5.   **Seated Tree Pose with Twist:** Start by sitting tall in your chair with your feet flat on the floor and your hands resting on your thighs. Inhale deeply, then exhale as you lift your right foot off the floor and place the sole of your right foot on your left inner thigh or calf, avoiding the knee. Inhale as you lengthen your spine, then exhale as you twist to the right, placing your left hand on your right knee and your right hand on the back of the chair. Hold for a few breaths, feeling the twist from your belly button all the way up to your shoulders. Inhale to release the twist, then exhale to return to center. Repeat on the other side. Seated Tree Pose with Twist improves balance, opens the chest, and stimulates digestion.

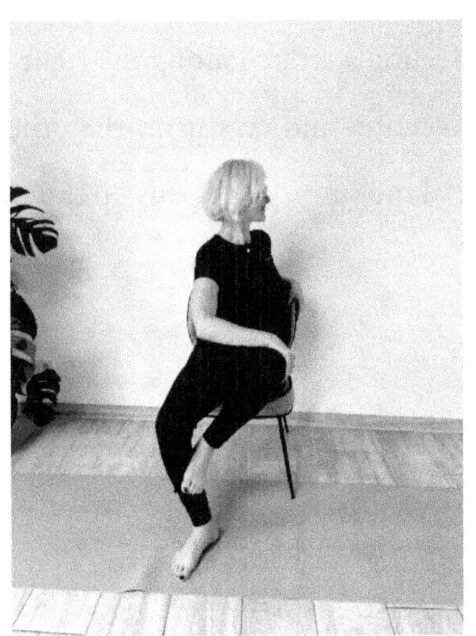 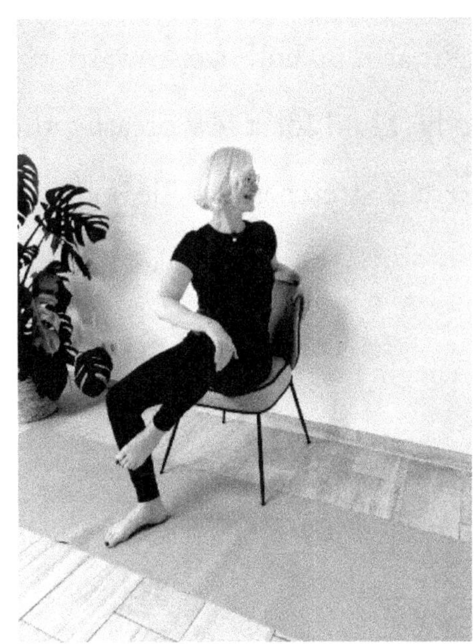

Day 2 - Day 9 – Day 16 – Day 23: Mobility Improvement

Today, I'm excited to share five intermediate-level exercises designed to enhance your mobility and improve your range of motion. Let's dive in!

Start your daily Yoga Routines with Breathwork and Warm-Up Exercises.

1. **Seated Side Stretch with Arm Reach:** Start by sitting tall in your chair with your feet flat on the floor and your hands resting on your thighs. Inhale deeply as you reach your right arm up and over towards the left side, feeling a stretch along the right side of your body. Hold for a few breaths, then return to center and repeat on the other side. This exercise stretches the side body, improves spinal mobility, and opens up the rib cage.

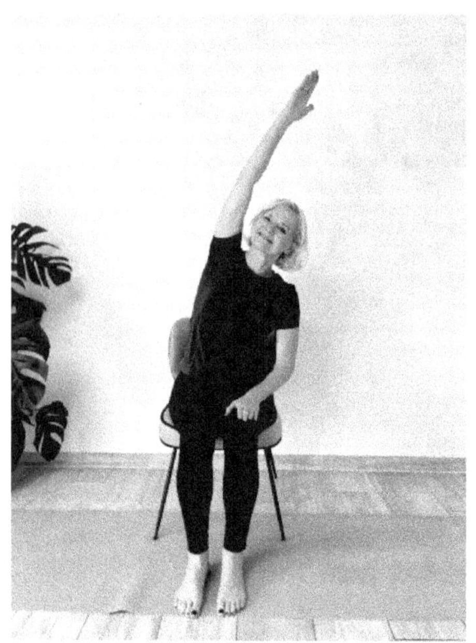 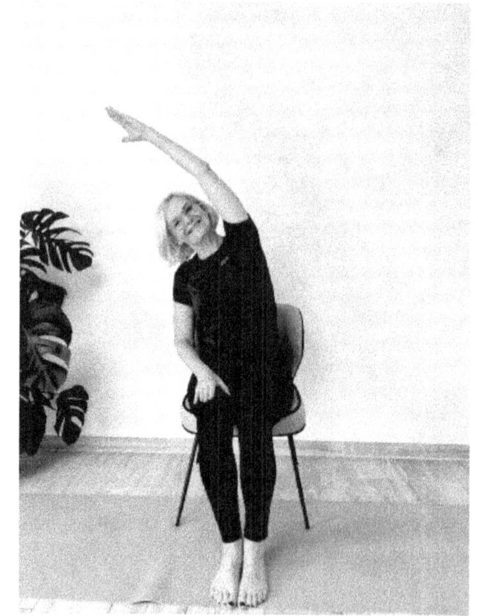

2. **Seated Figure Four Stretch:** Sit towards the front edge of your chair with your feet flat on the floor and your hands resting on your thighs. Cross your right ankle over your left knee, flexing your right foot to protect your knee. Inhale deeply as you lengthen your spine, then exhale as you hinge forward from your hips, bringing your chest towards your right shin. Hold for a few breaths, feeling a stretch in your right hip and glute. Repeat on the other side. This exercise improves hip mobility and flexibility.

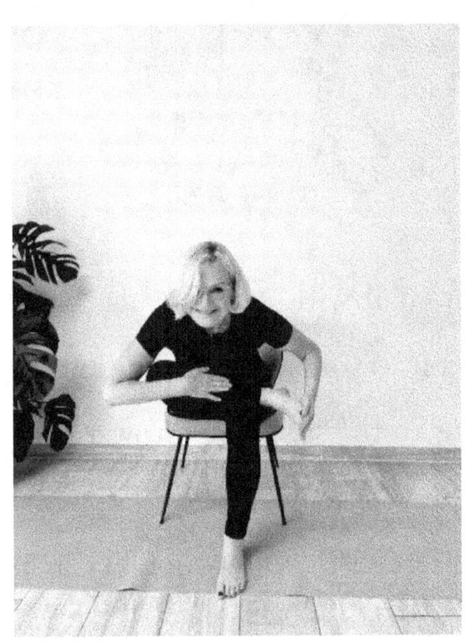 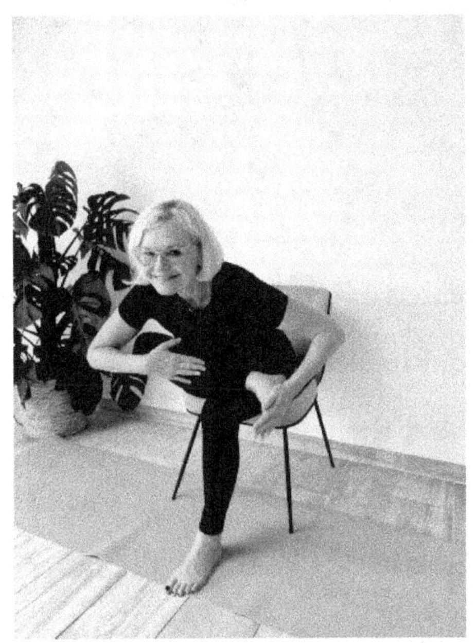

3. **Seated Knee-to-Chest Stretch:** Sit tall in your chair with your feet flat on the floor and your hands resting on your thighs. Inhale deeply, then exhale as you hug your right knee towards your chest, wrapping your arms around your shin. Hold for a few breaths, feeling a stretch in your right hip and lower back. Release and repeat on the other side. This exercise increases flexibility in the hips and relieves tension in the lower back.

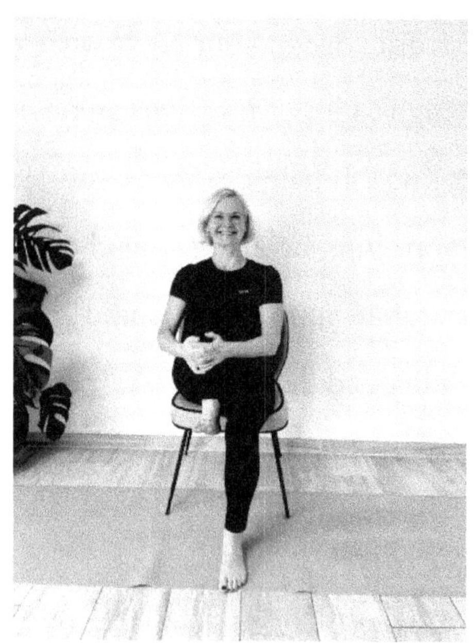 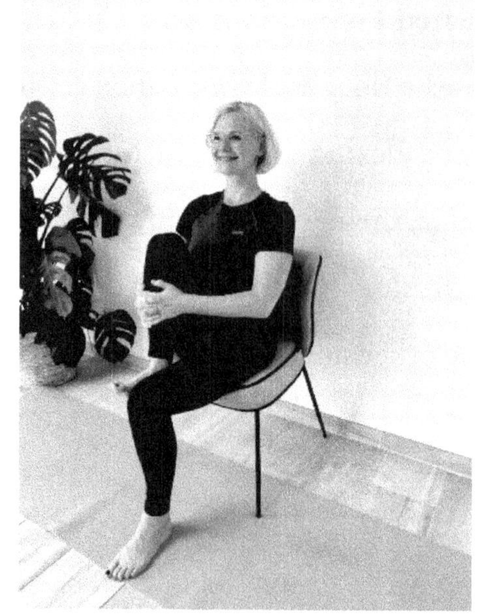

4. **Seated Hip Circles:** Sit comfortably in your chair with your feet flat on the floor and your hands resting on your thighs. Inhale deeply as you lift your right knee towards your chest, then exhale as you circle your knee out to the side, down towards the floor, and back up towards your chest. Repeat this circular motion several times, then switch directions. Repeat on the other side. This exercise increases mobility in the hips and improves circulation in the lower body.

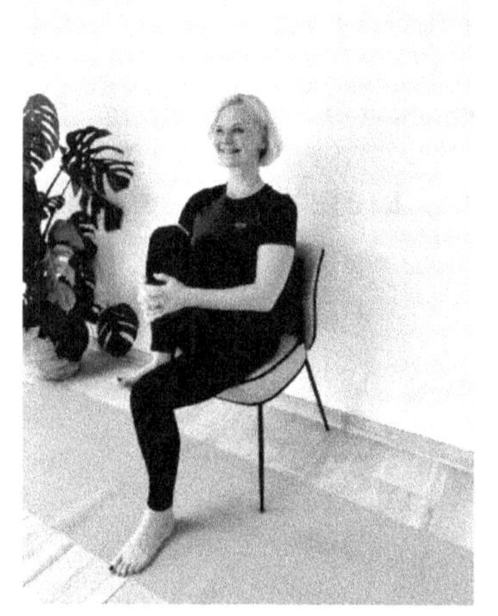 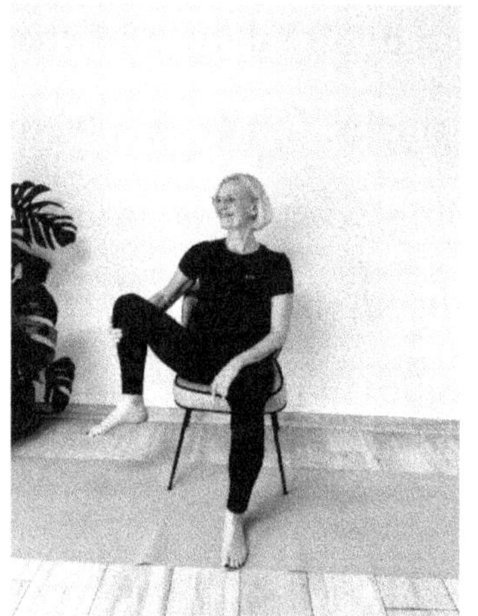 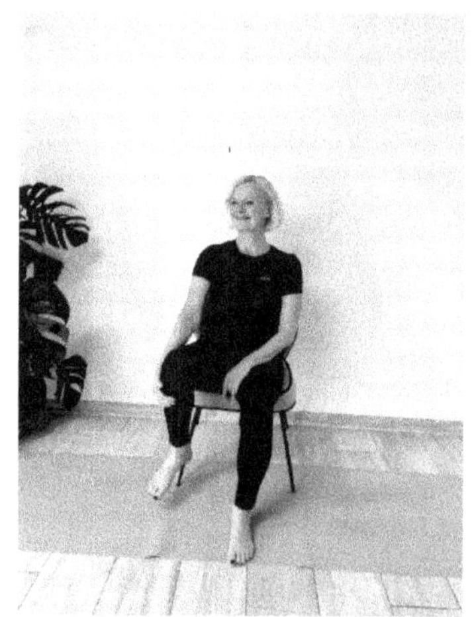

5. **Seated Neck Rolls:** Sit tall in your chair with your feet flat on the floor and your hands resting on your thighs. Inhale deeply as you lengthen your spine, then exhale as you drop your chin towards your chest, feeling a stretch in the back of your neck. Inhale as you roll your right ear towards your right shoulder, then exhale as you continue to roll your head back until your left ear reaches your left shoulder. Inhale to return to center, then exhale to repeat on the other side. This exercise releases tension in the neck and improves neck mobility.

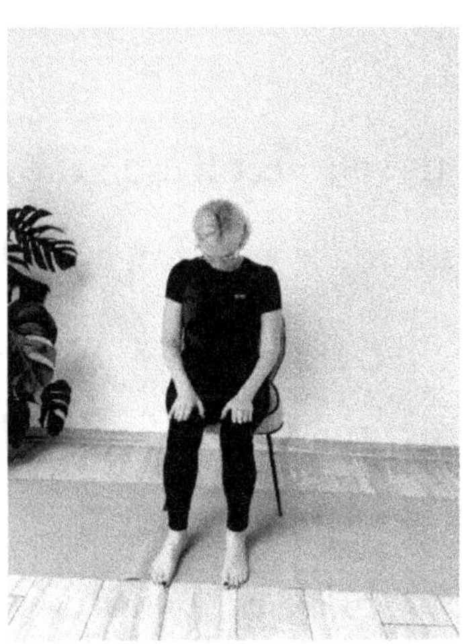
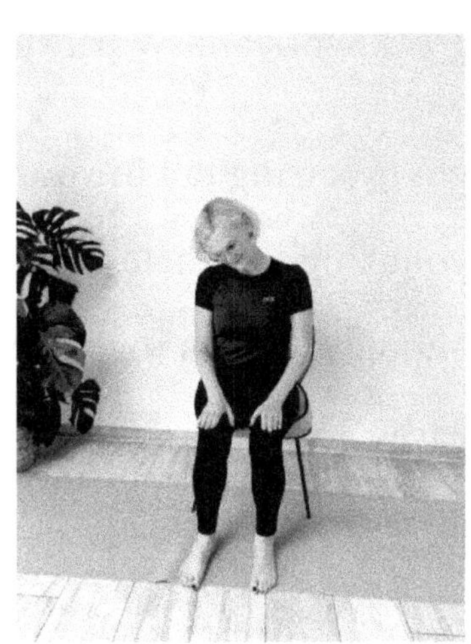
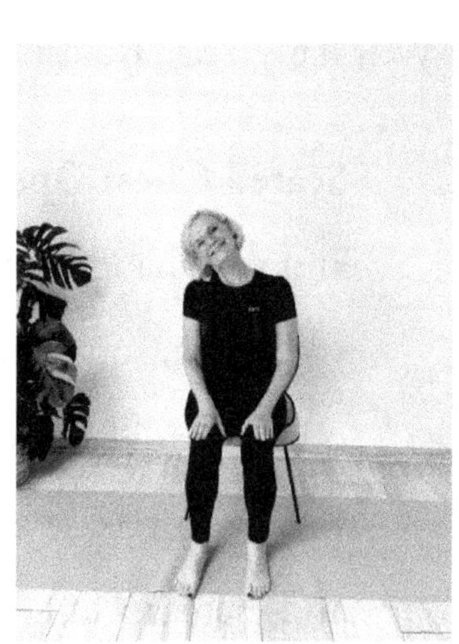

Day 3 – Day 10 – Day 17 – Day 24: Poses for Heart Health

Today, I'm thrilled to share five intermediate-level poses specifically designed to promote heart health and vitality. These exercises will help you strengthen your cardiovascular system, improve circulation, and boost your overall well-being. Let's get started!

Start your daily Yoga Routines with Breathwork and Warm-Up Exercises.

1. **Seated Chest Opener:** Begin by sitting tall in your chair with your feet flat on the floor and your hands resting on your thighs. Inhale deeply as you interlace your fingers behind your back, squeezing your shoulder blades together and opening your chest towards the ceiling. Hold for a few breaths, feeling a gentle stretch across the front of your chest. Exhale to release and repeat as desired. This pose improves posture, expands the chest, and increases lung capacity.

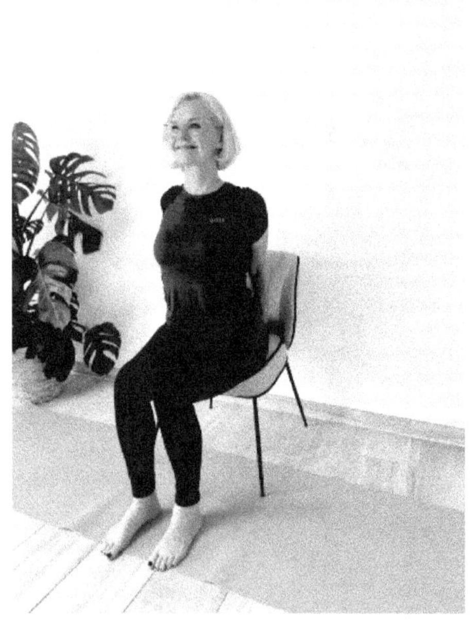
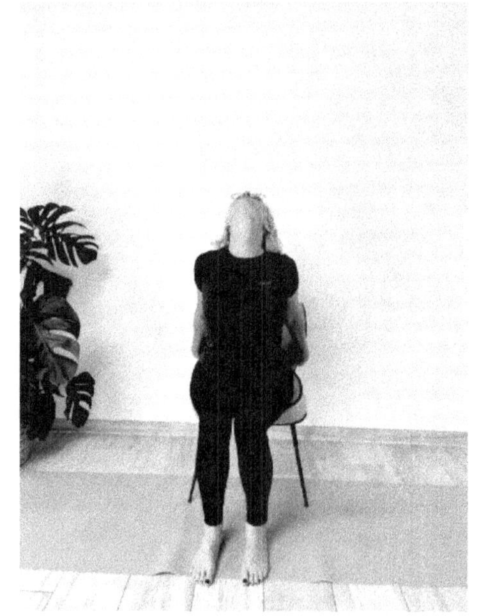

2. **Seated Backbend:** Sit towards the front edge of your chair with your feet flat on the floor and your hands resting on your thighs. Inhale deeply as you lift your chest towards the ceiling, arching your back slightly and drawing your shoulder blades together. Keep your neck long and relaxed. Hold for a few breaths, feeling a stretch along the front of your body. Exhale to release and repeat as desired. This pose opens the heart center, stimulates circulation, and boosts energy levels.

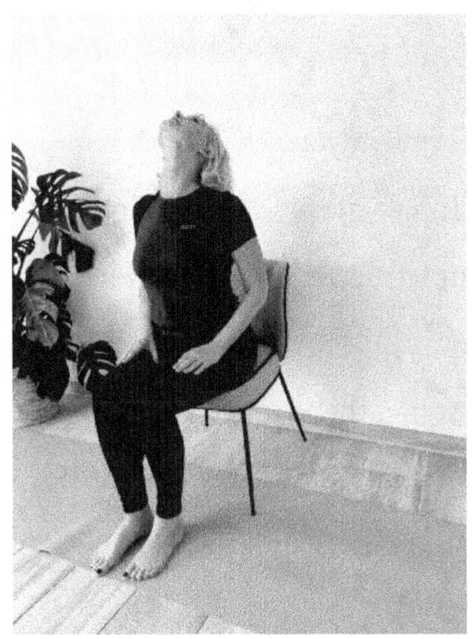

3. **Seated Forward Fold with Heart Mudra:** Sit tall in your chair with your feet flat on the floor and your hands resting on your thighs. Inhale deeply as you reach your arms overhead, lengthening your spine. Exhale as you hinge forward from your hips, bringing your chest towards your thighs and reaching your arms out in front of you. As you fold forward, bring the palms of your hands together in front of your heart in a prayer position. Hold for a few breaths, feeling a stretch along the spine and the back of the legs. This pose calms the mind, relieves stress, and opens the heart center.

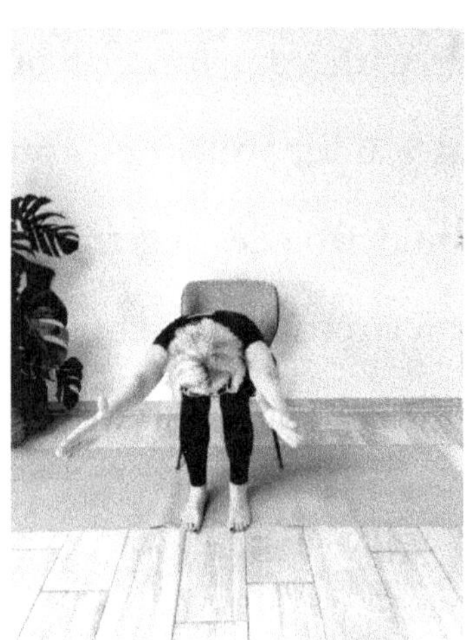 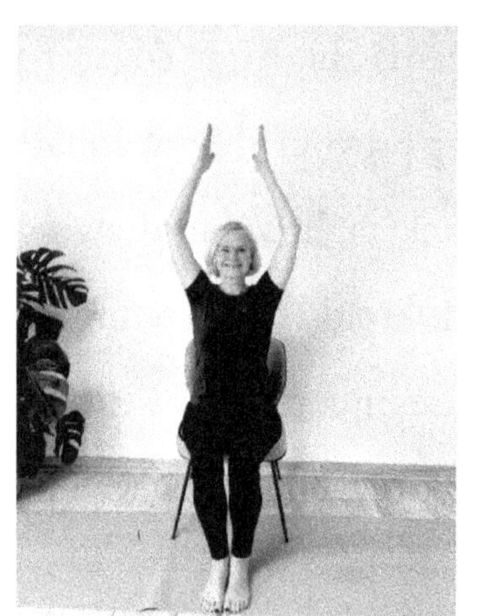 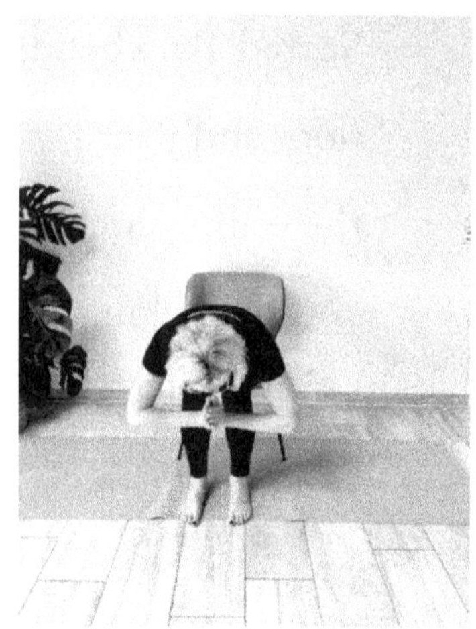

4.   **Seated Spinal Twist:** Sit tall in your chair with your feet flat on the floor and your hands resting on your thighs. Inhale deeply as you lengthen your spine, then exhale as you twist to the right, placing your left hand on the outside of your right knee and your right hand on the back of the chair. Hold for a few breaths, feeling a gentle twist along the spine. Inhale to lengthen the spine, then exhale to deepen the twist. Repeat on the other side. This pose improves digestion, stimulates the cardiovascular system, and detoxifies the body.

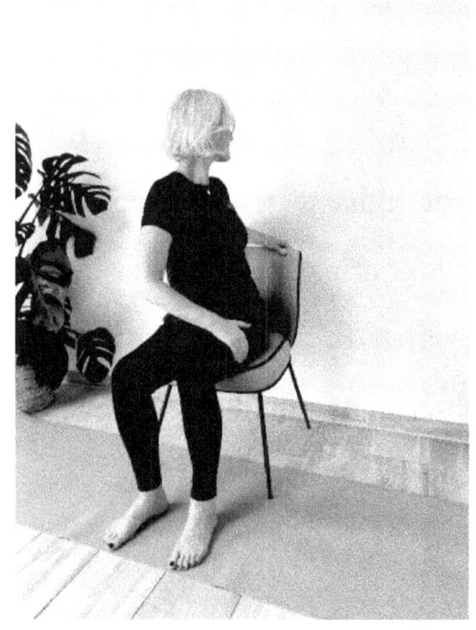 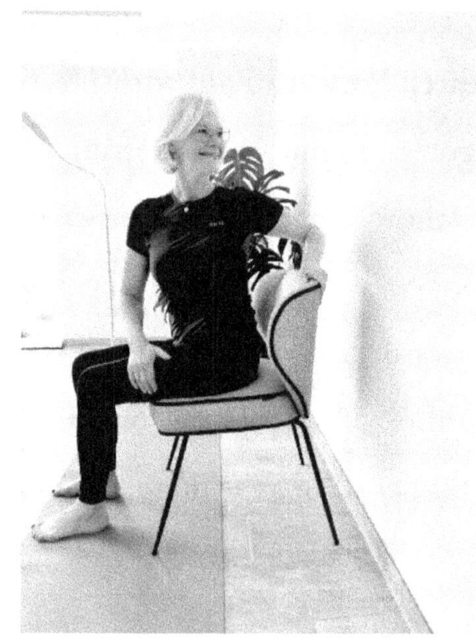

5. **Seated Camel Pose:** Sit towards the front edge of your chair with your feet flat on the floor and your hands resting on your thighs. Inhale deeply as you lift your chest towards the ceiling, arching your back and bringing your hands to rest on the back of the chair. Keep your neck long and relaxed. Hold for a few breaths, feeling a stretch across the front of your body. Exhale to release and repeat as desired. This pose strengthens the back muscles, opens the chest, and promotes heart health.

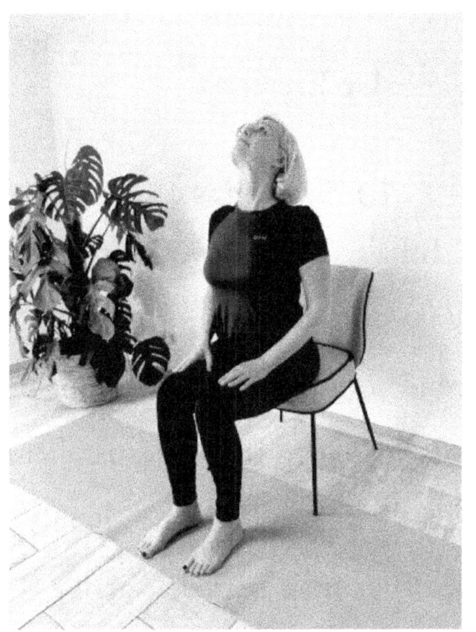 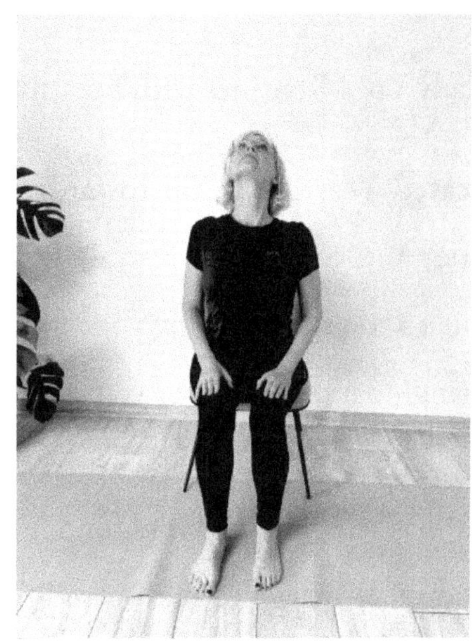

Day 4 – Day 11 – Day 18 – Day 25: Building Strength

Are you ready to build strength and resilience in your practice? Today, I'm excited to share intermediate-level exercises designed to help you increase muscle tone, improve stability, and enhance your overall strength. Let's dive in!

Start your daily Yoga Routines with Breathwork and Warm-Up Exercises.

1. **Seated Warrior II:** Sit towards the front edge of your chair with your feet flat on the floor and your hands resting on your thighs. Inhale deeply as you extend your right leg out to the side, keeping your foot flat on the floor. Exhale as you bend your right knee, bringing it directly over your right ankle. Extend your left leg out behind you, keeping it straight and strong. Inhale as you reach your arms out to the sides, parallel to the floor, palms facing down. Hold for a few breaths, feeling the strength and stability in your legs and core. Exhale to release and repeat on the other side. Seated Warrior II strengthens the legs, opens the hips, and improves balance.

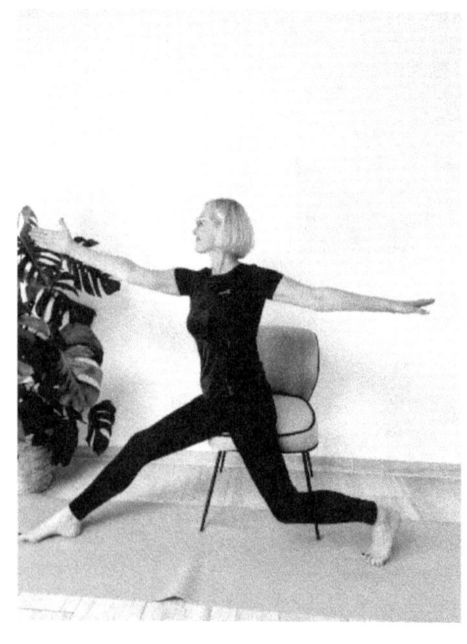
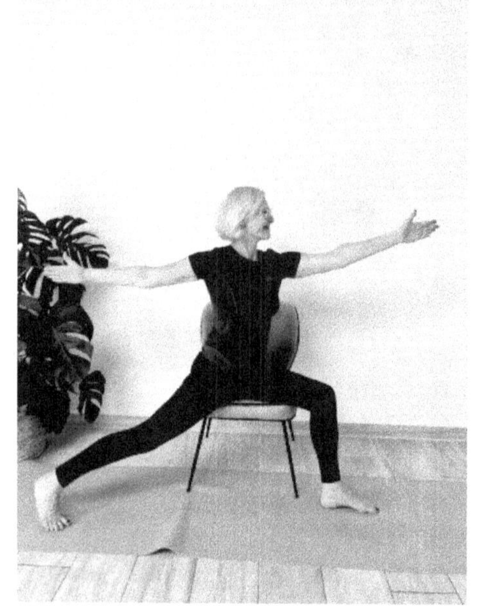

2. **Seated Chair Pose with Twist:** Start by sitting tall in your chair with your feet flat on the floor and your hands resting on your thighs. Inhale deeply as you lift your arms overhead, palms facing each other. Exhale as you bend your elbows and bring your hands together in prayer position. Inhale to lengthen your spine, then exhale as you twist to the right, placing your left elbow on the outside of your right knee and your right hand on the back of the chair. Hold for a few breaths, feeling the engagement in your core and the stretch in your spine. Inhale to return to center, then exhale to repeat on the other side. Seated Chair Pose with Twist strengthens the core, improves digestion, and detoxifies the body.

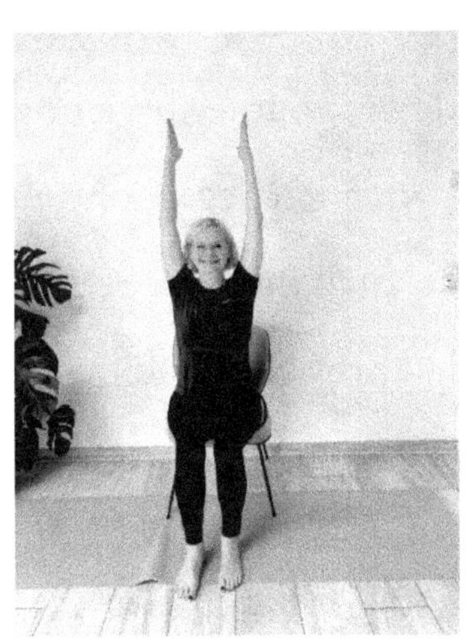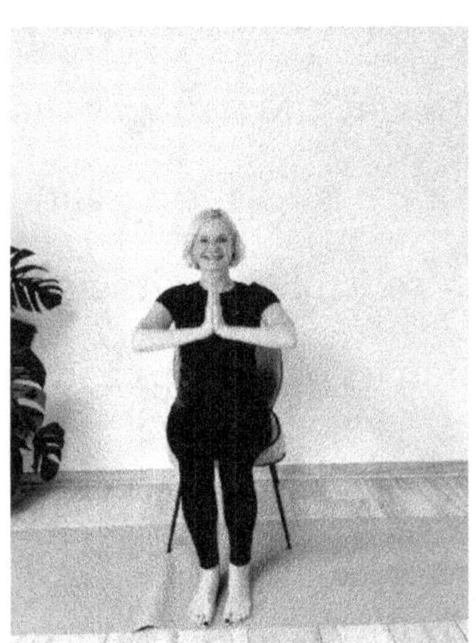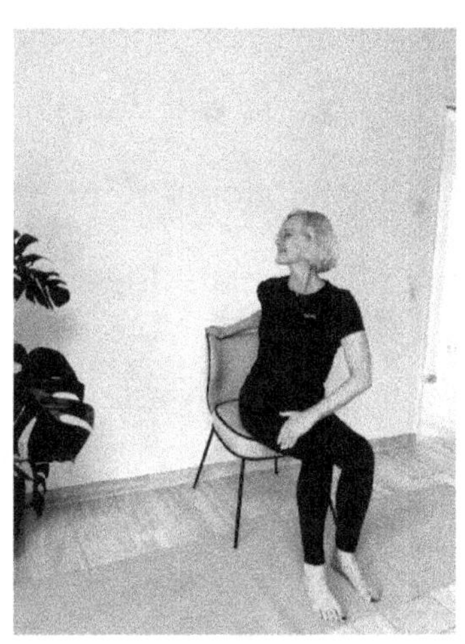

3. **Seated Leg Press:** Sit tall in your chair with your feet flat on the floor and your hands resting on your thighs. Inhale deeply as you lift your right foot off the floor, bringing your knee towards your chest. Exhale as you extend your right leg out in front of you, pressing through your heel. Hold for a few breaths, feeling the engagement in your quadriceps and hamstrings. Inhale to bend your knee and bring your foot back to the floor. Repeat on the other side. Seated Leg Press strengthens the muscles of the legs and improves lower body strength and stability.

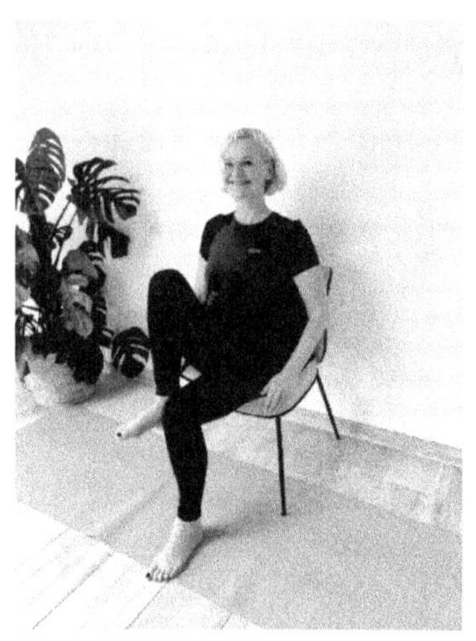 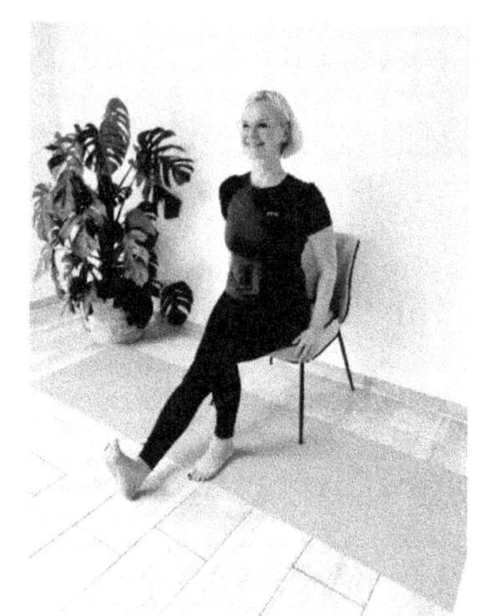 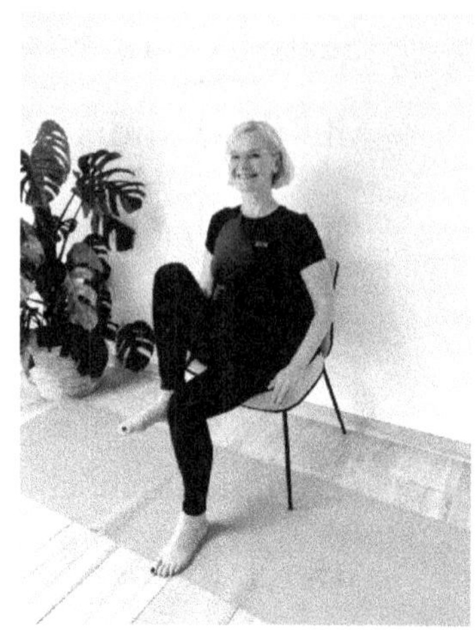

4. **Seated Side Leg Raises:** Sit towards the front edge of your chair with your feet flat on the floor and your hands resting on your thighs. Inhale deeply as you lift your right leg out to the side, keeping it straight and strong. Exhale as you lower your leg back down to the floor. Repeat on the other side, lifting and lowering your left leg. Continue to alternate sides, moving with control and engaging your outer thigh muscles. Seated Side Leg Raises strengthen the muscles of the hips and thighs and improve hip stability.

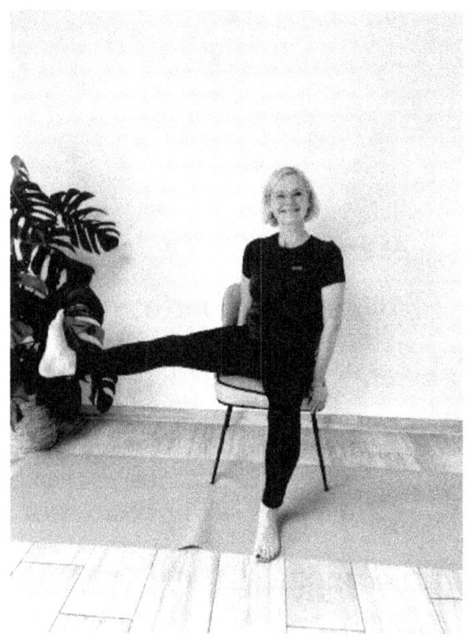 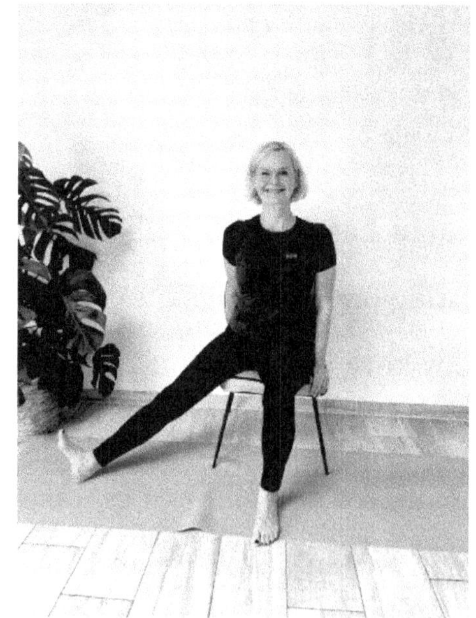

5. **Seated Shoulder Press:** Sit tall in your chair with your feet flat on the floor and your hands resting on your thighs. Inhale deeply as you lift your arms out to the sides, palms facing forward. Exhale as you press your arms overhead, reaching towards the ceiling. Hold for a few breaths, feeling the engagement in your shoulder muscles. Inhale to lower your arms back down to shoulder height, then exhale to repeat. Seated Shoulder Press strengthens the muscles of the shoulders, arms, and upper back, improving posture and upper body strength.

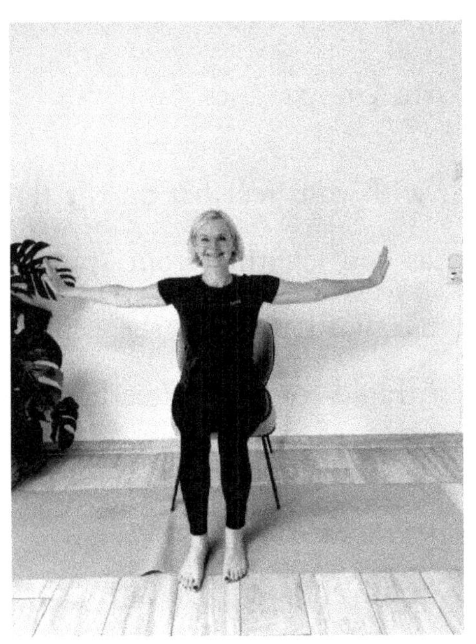
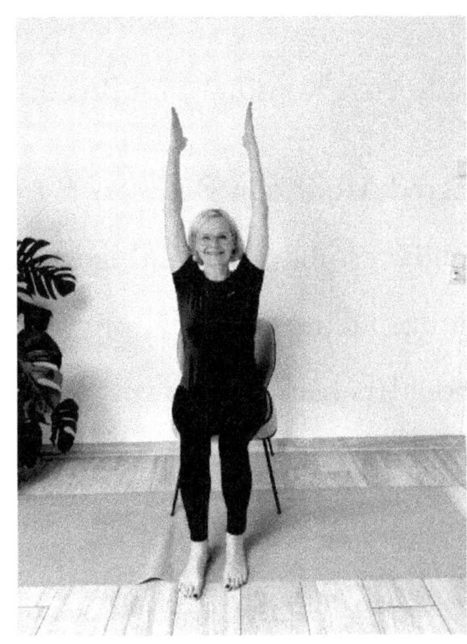

Day 5 – Day 12 – Day 19 – Day 26: Improved Posture and Alignment

Today, I'm excited to share five intermediate-level exercises designed to help you improve your posture and alignment, supporting a strong and healthy spine. These exercises will help you cultivate greater awareness of your body and maintain proper alignment throughout your practice. Let's dive in!

Start your daily Yoga Routines with Breathwork and Warm-Up Exercises.

1. **Seated Mountain Pose:** Sit tall in your chair with your feet flat on the floor and your hands resting on your thighs. Inhale deeply as you lengthen your spine, imagining a string pulling you up from the crown of your head towards the ceiling. Roll your shoulders back and down, opening your chest. Hold for a few breaths, feeling tall and aligned. Seated Mountain Pose helps to improve posture by lengthening the spine and promoting proper alignment.

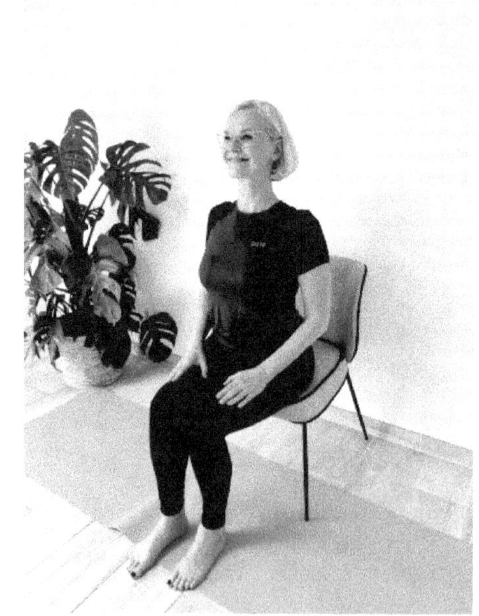

2. **Seated Shoulder Blade Squeeze:** Sit tall in your chair with your feet flat on the floor and your hands resting on your thighs. Inhale deeply as you squeeze your shoulder blades together behind you, opening your chest and drawing your shoulders back. Hold for a few breaths, feeling the muscles between your shoulder blades engage. Exhale to release and repeat as desired. Seated Shoulder Blade Squeeze strengthens the muscles of the upper back and improves posture by promoting scapular retraction.

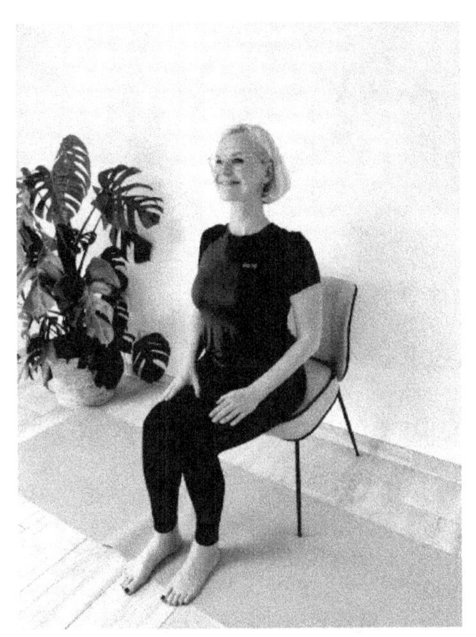 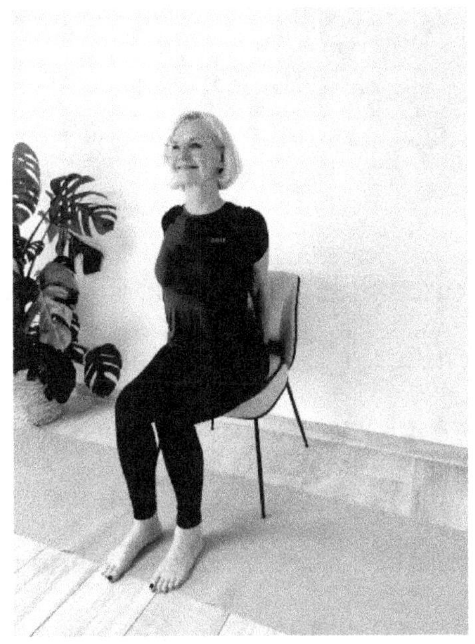

3. **Seated Chest Expansion:** Sit towards the front edge of your chair with your feet flat on the floor and your hands resting on your thighs. Inhale deeply as you interlace your fingers behind your back, straightening your arms and lifting your chest towards the ceiling. Draw your shoulder blades together and down, opening your chest wide. Hold for a few breaths, feeling a stretch across the front of your chest. Exhale to release and repeat as desired. Seated Chest Expansion helps to counteract the effects of slouching and promotes an open and expansive posture.

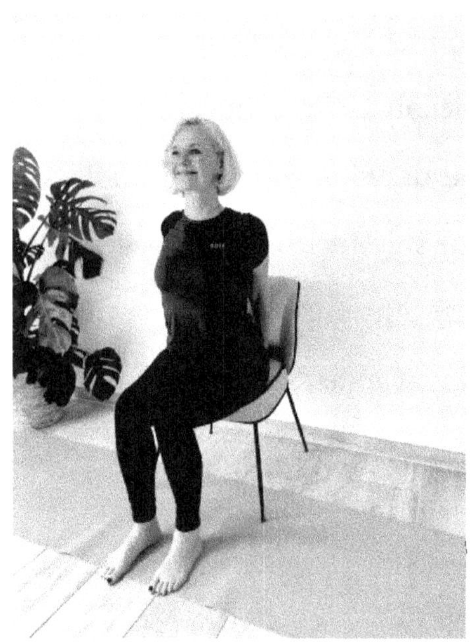 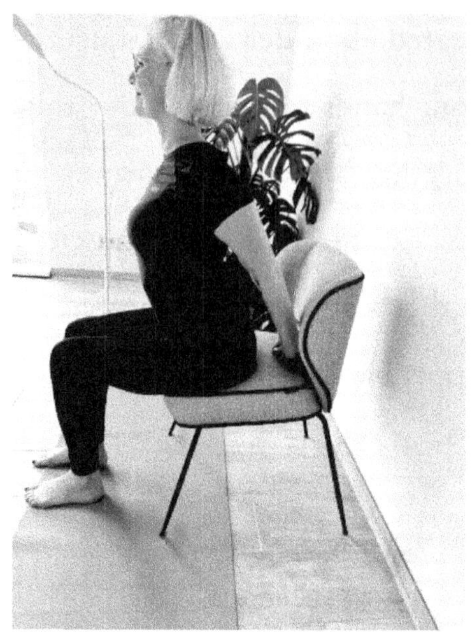

4. **Seated Side Stretch:** Sit tall in your chair with your feet flat on the floor and your hands resting on your thighs. Inhale deeply as you reach your right arm up and over towards the left side, creating a long line of energy from your right fingertips to your right hip. Keep both sit bones grounded on the chair and your left hand resting gently on your left thigh. Hold for a few breaths, feeling a stretch along the right side of your body. Exhale to release and repeat on the other side. Seated Side Stretch helps to lengthen the muscles along the sides of the body and improve lateral flexibility.

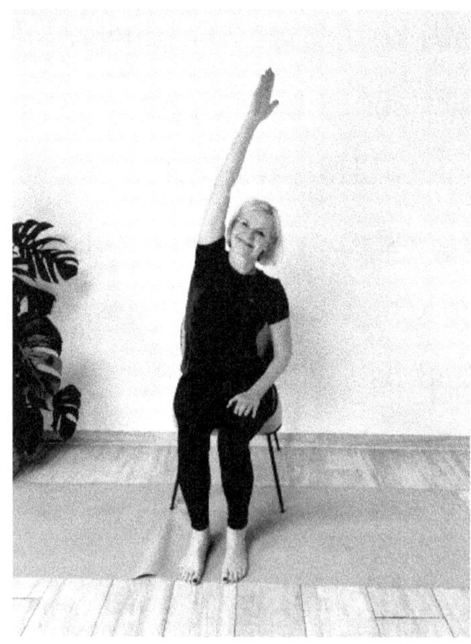

5. **Seated Core Activation:** Sit tall in your chair with your feet flat on the floor and your hands resting on your thighs. Inhale deeply as you engage your core muscles, drawing your navel towards your spine and lifting your chest towards the ceiling. Hold for a few breaths, feeling a gentle activation of the muscles around your abdomen and lower back. Exhale to release and repeat as desired. Seated Core Activation helps to strengthen the muscles of the core and improve posture by providing support to the spine.

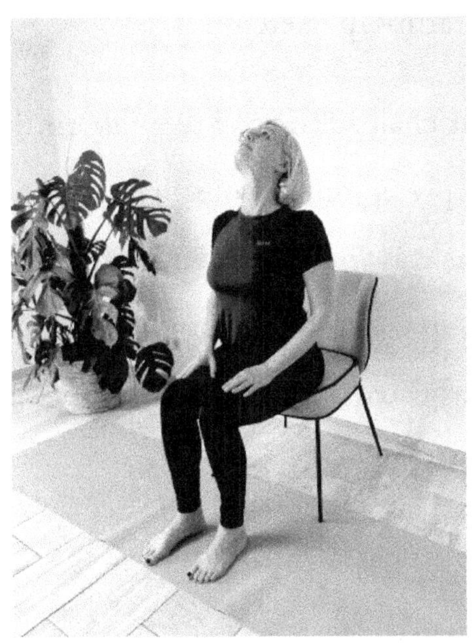
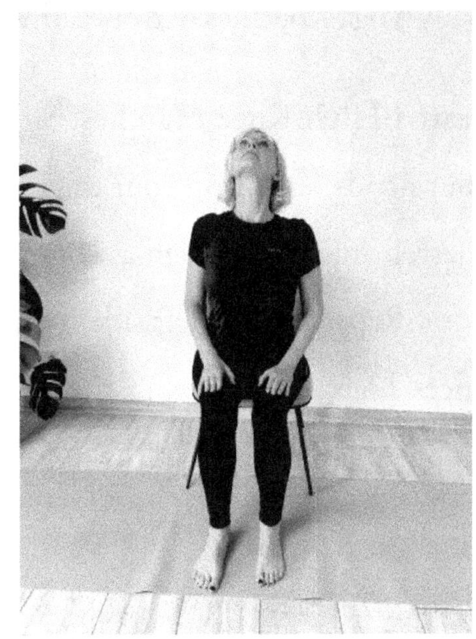

Day 6 – Day 13 – Day 20 – Day 27: Mobility and Strength

Today, I'm excited to share five additional exercises for improving mobility and strength in Chair Yoga for intermediate seniors:

Start your daily Yoga Routines with Breathwork and Warm-Up Exercises.

1. **Seated High Knee Marches**: Sit tall in your chair with your feet flat on the floor and your hands resting on your thighs. Inhale deeply as you lift your right knee towards your chest, bringing it as high as comfortable. Exhale as you lower your right foot back to the floor. Repeat on the left side, alternating legs in a marching motion. Focus on lifting the knees high and engaging the core muscles. Seated High Knee Marches improve hip mobility and strengthen the muscles of the lower body.

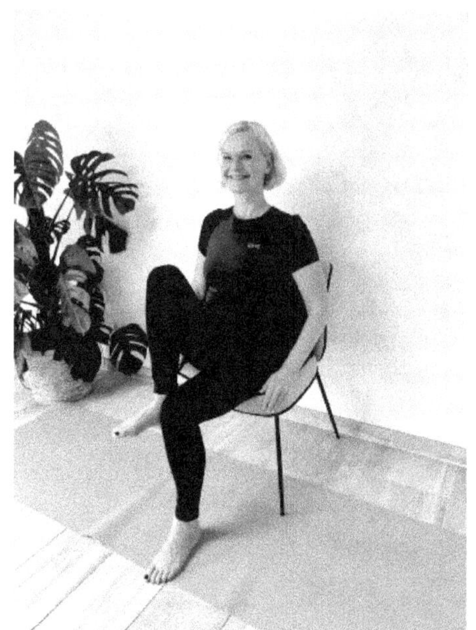

2. **Seated Leg Circles:** Sit towards the front edge of your chair with your feet flat on the floor and your hands resting on your thighs. Inhale deeply as you lift your right foot off the floor, extending your leg out in front of you. Exhale as you make small circles with your right foot, moving clockwise for several repetitions, then counterclockwise. Repeat on the left side. Seated Leg Circles improve hip mobility, increase circulation, and strengthen the muscles of the legs.

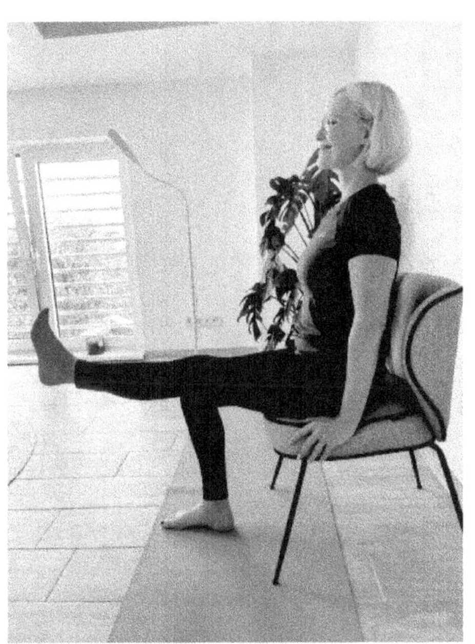 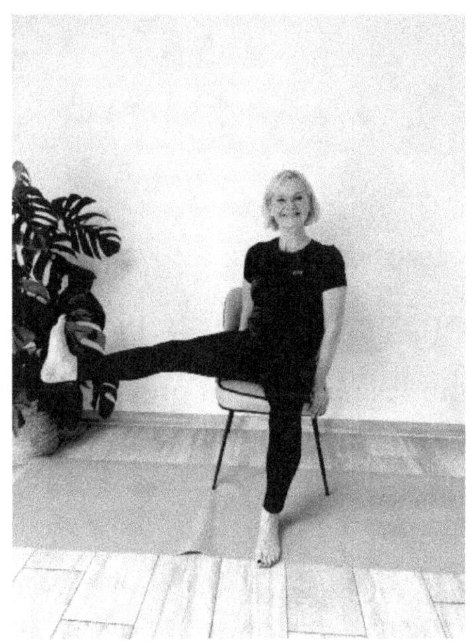

3. **Seated Side Leg Lifts with Resistance Band:** Sit tall in your chair with your feet flat on the floor and a resistance band looped around your thighs, just above your knees. Inhale deeply as you press your knees out against the resistance of the band, engaging the muscles of the outer thighs. Exhale as you release the tension and bring your knees back to center. Repeat for several repetitions, focusing on the outward movement. Seated Side Leg Lifts with Resistance Band strengthen the muscles of the outer thighs and hips, improving hip stability and mobility.

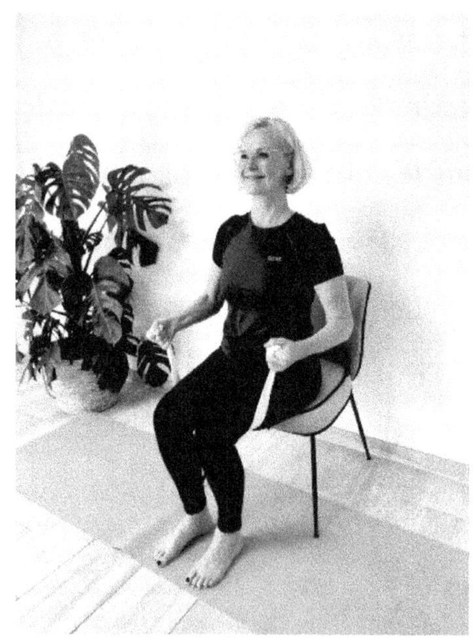

4. **Seated Toe Taps:** Sit tall in your chair with your feet flat on the floor and your hands resting on your thighs. Inhale deeply as you lift your right foot off the floor, extending your leg out in front of you. Exhale as you tap your right toes lightly on the floor in front of you, then lift your foot back up. Repeat for several repetitions, then switch to the left side. Seated Toe Taps improve ankle mobility, strengthen the muscles of the legs, and promote balance.

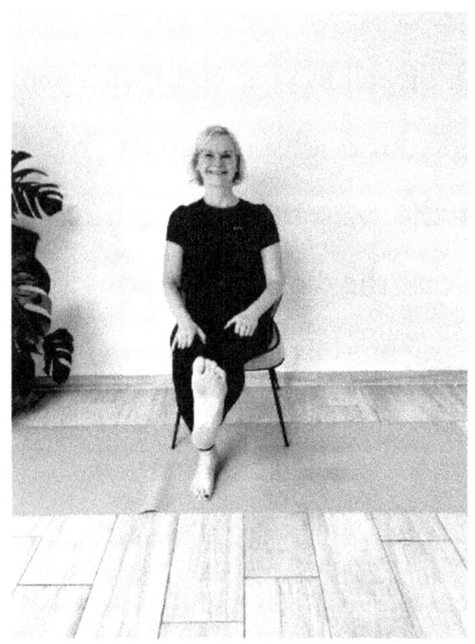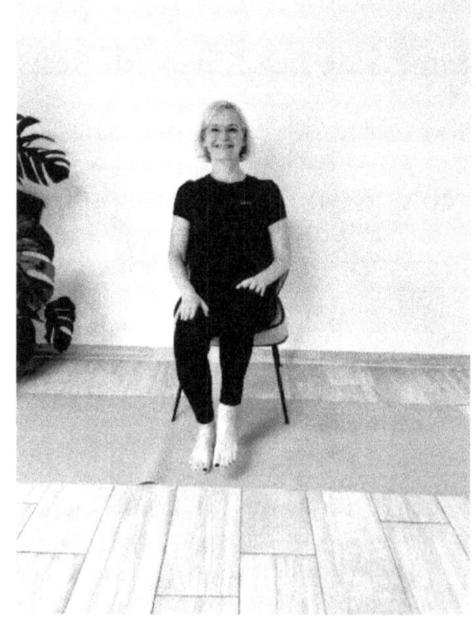

5. **Seated Hip Openers:** Sit towards the front edge of your chair with your feet flat on the floor and your hands resting on your thighs. Inhale deeply as you lift your right foot off the floor, placing your right ankle on top of your left knee in a figure-four position. Exhale as you gently press down on your right knee, opening up the hip. Hold for a few breaths, feeling a stretch in the outer hip and thigh. Release and repeat on the other side. Seated Hip Openers improve hip mobility, reduce tension in the hips, and strengthen the muscles of the legs.

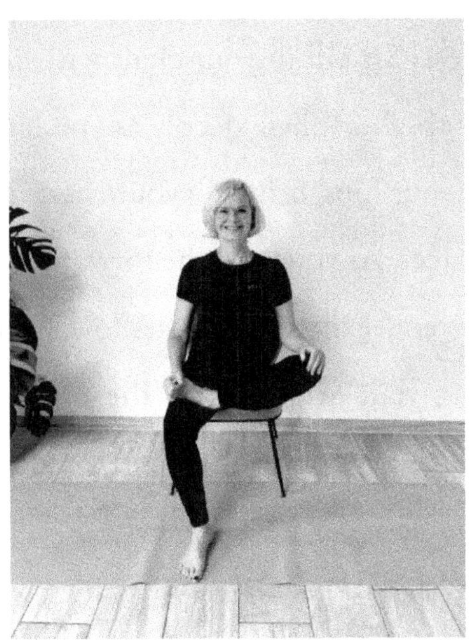 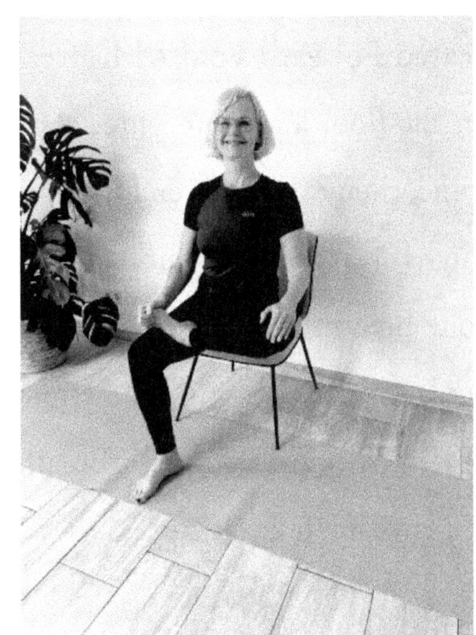

Day 7 – Day 14 – Day 21 – Day 28: Enhanced Mental Clarity and Focus

As we embark on our Chair Yoga journey, let's explore five additional exercises for enhancing mental clarity and focus in Chair Yoga for intermediate seniors:

Start your daily Yoga Routines with Breathwork and Warm-Up Exercises.

1. **Seated Forward Fold with Breath Awareness:** Sit tall in your chair with your feet flat on the floor and your hands resting on your thighs. Inhale deeply as you lengthen your spine, then exhale as you hinge forward from your hips, bringing your chest towards your thighs and reaching your hands towards your feet. As you hold the forward fold, focus on your breath, inhaling deeply into your belly and exhaling fully. Allow your breath to guide you deeper into the stretch and bring your attention to the present moment. Seated Forward Fold with Breath Awareness helps to calm the mind, reduce stress, and improve mental clarity.

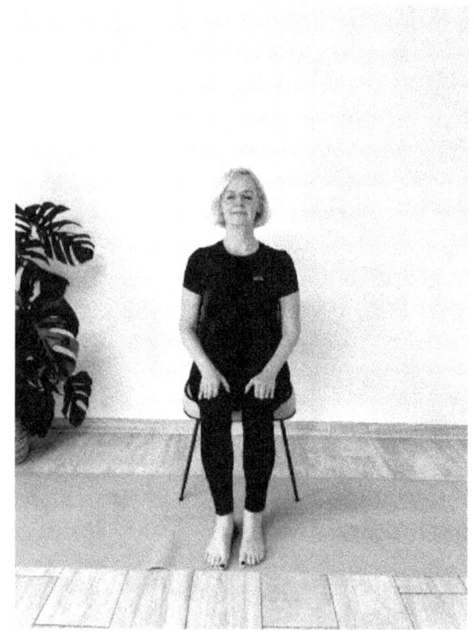
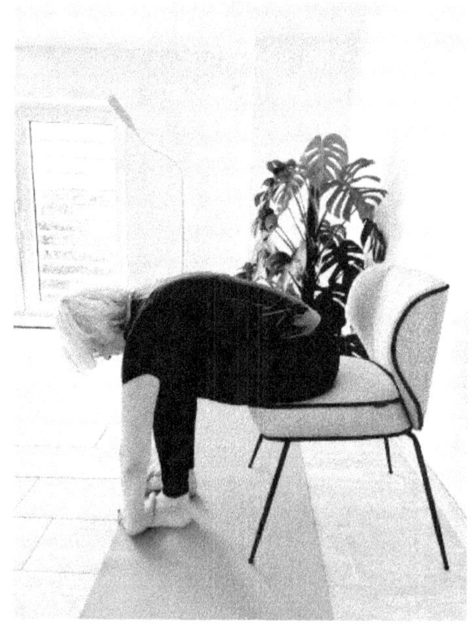

2. **Seated Eagle Arms with Visualization:** Sit tall in your chair with your feet flat on the floor and your hands resting on your thighs. Inhale deeply as you reach your arms out to the sides, then exhale as you cross your right arm under your left arm, bringing your palms together in front of your face. As you hold the eagle arms, visualize yourself soaring high above, feeling a sense of freedom and expansiveness. Focus on the sensation of openness and release any tension or tightness in your body. Seated Eagle Arms with Visualization helps to quiet the mind, promote relaxation, and enhance mental clarity.

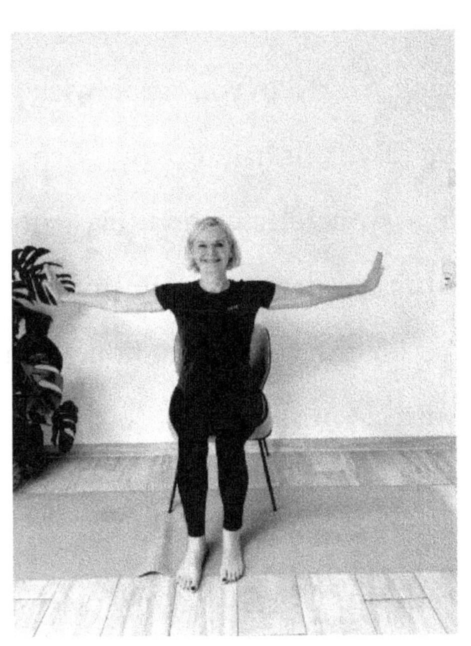 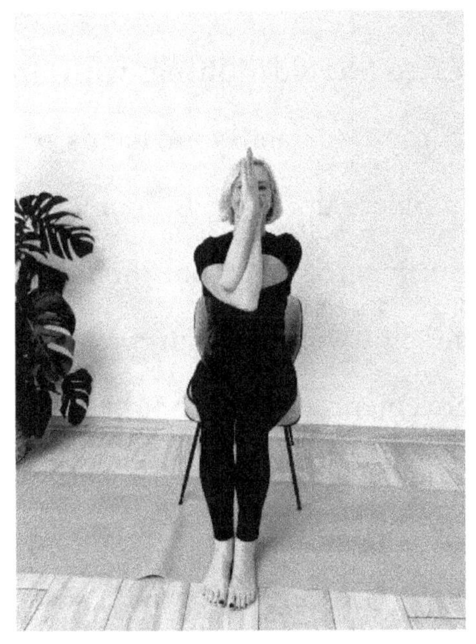

3. **Seated Neck Rolls with Affirmations:** Sit tall in your chair with your feet flat on the floor and your hands resting on your thighs. Inhale deeply as you gently drop your chin towards your chest, then exhale as you roll your head to the right, bringing your right ear towards your right shoulder. As you hold the stretch, repeat a positive affirmation to yourself, such as "I am calm and focused" or "My mind is clear and sharp." Inhale to return to center, then exhale to repeat on the left side. Seated Neck Rolls with Affirmations helps to release tension in the neck and shoulders, promote positive thinking, and improve mental clarity.

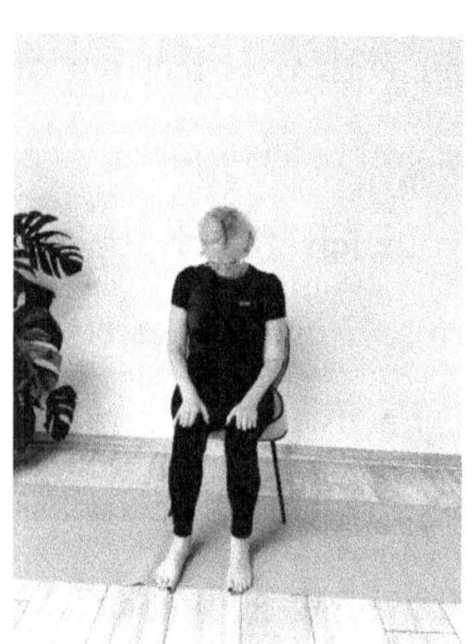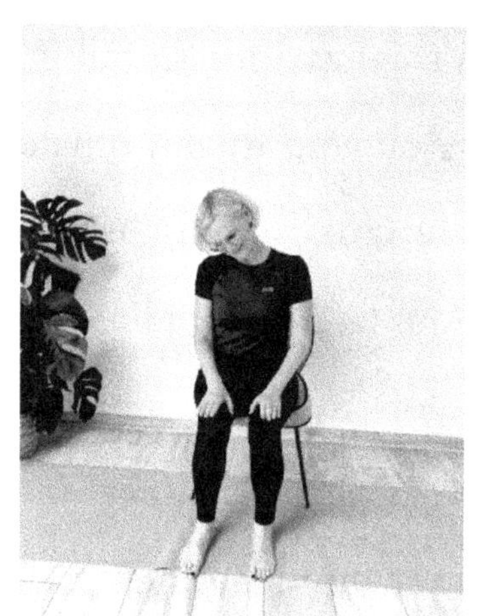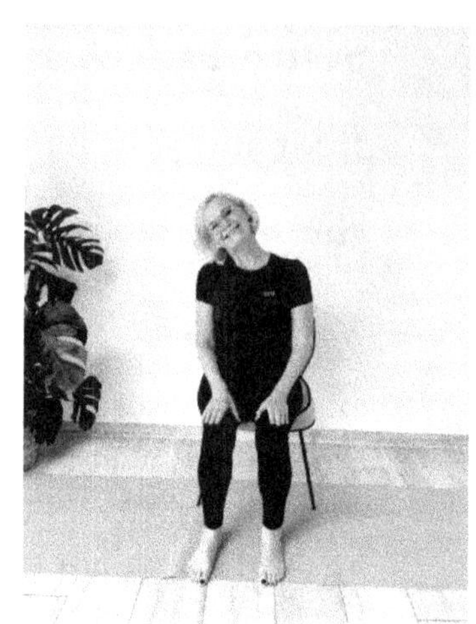

4. **Seated Shoulder Shrugs with Breath Counting**: Sit tall in your chair with your feet flat on the floor and your hands resting on your thighs. Inhale deeply as you shrug your shoulders up towards your ears, then exhale as you release them back down. As you continue to shrug your shoulders, count each breath silently in your mind, starting from one and working your way up to five. Focus on the rhythm of your breath and the movement of your shoulders, allowing any distracting thoughts to float away. Seated Shoulder Shrugs with Breath Counting helps to release tension in the shoulders, promote mindfulness, and improve mental focus.

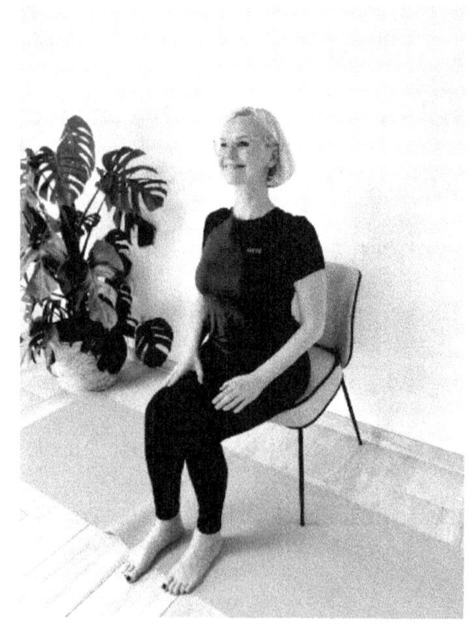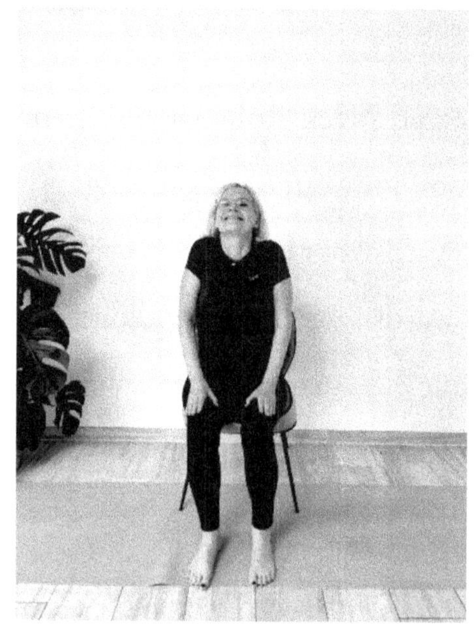

5. **Seated Twist and Release with Mantra:** Sit tall in your chair with your feet flat on the floor and your hands resting on your thighs. Inhale deeply as you lengthen your spine, then exhale as you twist to the right, placing your left hand on the outside of your right knee and your right hand on the back of the chair. As you hold the twist, silently repeat a calming mantra to yourself, such as "I am centered and grounded" or "I trust in the wisdom of my body." Inhale to return to center, then exhale to repeat on the left side. Seated Twist and Release with Mantra helps to improve digestion, release tension in the spine, and enhance mental clarity.

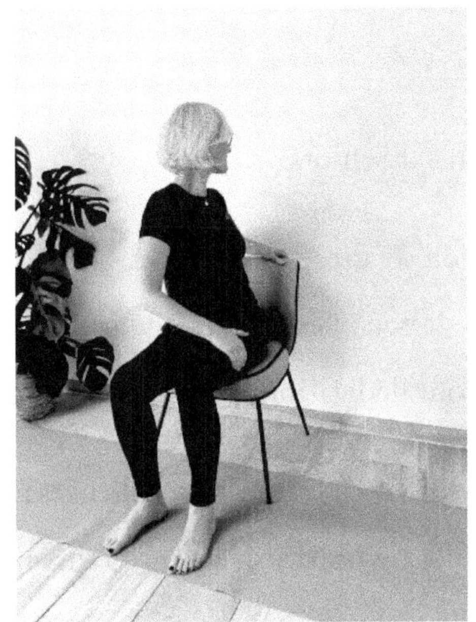 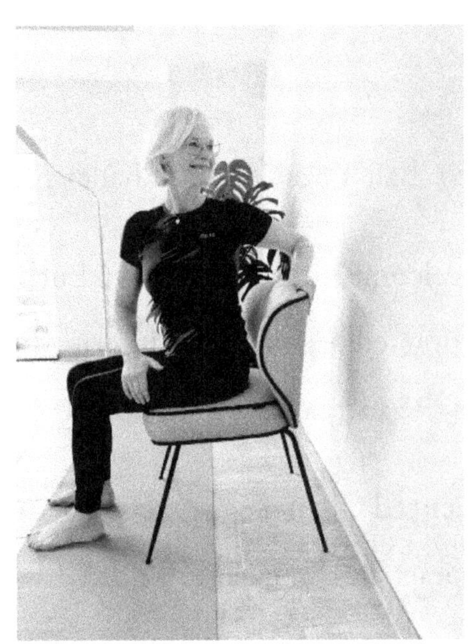

We'll see you in the next level! Keep up the fantastic work!

PART 6

Chair Yoga for Advanced

Welcome to Chair Yoga 28-Day Challenge for Experienced Seniors.

Hello and welcome, dear Chair Yoga Enthusiasts! If you've already embarked on the Chair Yoga journey, completed beginner and intermediate levels, or if you're exceptionally fit and ready to dive straight into the advanced course, I commend you for your dedication to health and well-being.

As an experienced Chair Yoga practitioner myself, I understand the unique challenges and joys that come with practicing yoga later in life. It's a journey filled with discovery, growth, and profound connection with our bodies and minds.

In this 28-day challenge, we'll delve deeper into the practice of Chair Yoga, exploring advanced poses, refining our techniques, and cultivating a deeper sense of awareness and mindfulness. Whether you're looking to enhance your strength, flexibility, or mental clarity, Chair Yoga offers a safe and accessible way to achieve your goals.

Throughout this journey, I'll be your guide, drawing upon my years of experience and understanding to support you every step of the way. But remember, yoga is ultimately a personal journey, and each of us will experience it in our own unique way.

So, as we embark on this adventure together, I encourage you to approach each practice with an open heart and a curious mind. Embrace the challenges, celebrate the victories, and above all, be kind to yourself.

Thank you for joining me on this journey. Together, let's explore the boundless potential of Chair Yoga and unlock the true essence of health, vitality, and inner peace.

So, roll out your mat, take a seat in your favorite chair, and get ready to embark on a journey of self-discovery and transformation through the practice of Chair Yoga.

28-Day Chair Yoga Challenge for Advanced

Dear Fellow Chair Yoga Enthusiast, as someone who has dedicated countless hours to honing my craft and sharing the benefits of Chair Yoga with others, I understand the transformative power of consistent practice and dedication.

To kickstart our journey together, I've curated seven meticulously detailed exercises designed to challenge and inspire you. These exercises are carefully crafted to build upon the foundation of strength, flexibility, and mindfulness that you've already cultivated, pushing you to new heights of physical and mental acuity.

But the real magic happens with repetition. After completing these initial exercises, I encourage you to commit to practicing them diligently for the next three weeks. Through repetition, you'll not only solidify your understanding of the movements but also refine them with greater precision and grace. Each repetition will bring you closer to mastery, making the movements feel more intuitive, effortless, and deeply satisfying.

But Chair Yoga isn't just about physical prowess—it's also about cultivating a sense of inner peace and tranquility. As you engage in these exercises, I invite you to connect with your breath, quiet your mind, and listen to the wisdom of your body. With each practice session, you'll deepen your sense of mindfulness and find yourself becoming more centered, grounded, and serene.

Through consistency and dedication, you'll not only enhance your physical strength and mobility but also cultivate a deeper sense of joy and fulfillment in your life. So, keep showing up on your mat, keep exploring, and keep growing. The rewards of your efforts will be undeniable, and you'll emerge from this challenge stronger, more agile, and with a renewed sense of peace and tranquility in your mind.

Remember, the journey of yoga is not about perfection but about progress. Embrace each moment, cherish each breath, and celebrate every small victory along the way.

Wishing you strength, mobility, and a peaceful mind on your Chair Yoga journey.

Day 1 – Day 8 – Day 15 – Day 22: Foundation Building Exercises for Balance

Incorporate these foundation-building exercises into your Chair Yoga practice to strengthen your body, improve flexibility, and enhance overall well-being. Remember to listen to your body and modify the poses as needed to suit your individual needs and abilities.

Start your daily Yoga Routines with Breathwork and Warm-Up Exercises.

1. **Seated Mountain Pose (Tadasana):** Sit tall in your chair with your feet flat on the floor and your hands resting on your thighs. Close your eyes and take a few deep breaths, feeling rooted and grounded like a mountain. Engage your core muscles and lengthen your spine, lifting your chest and rolling your shoulders back. Hold the pose for several breaths, focusing on your alignment and stability. Seated Mountain Pose helps to strengthen the foundation of your practice, improving posture and balance.

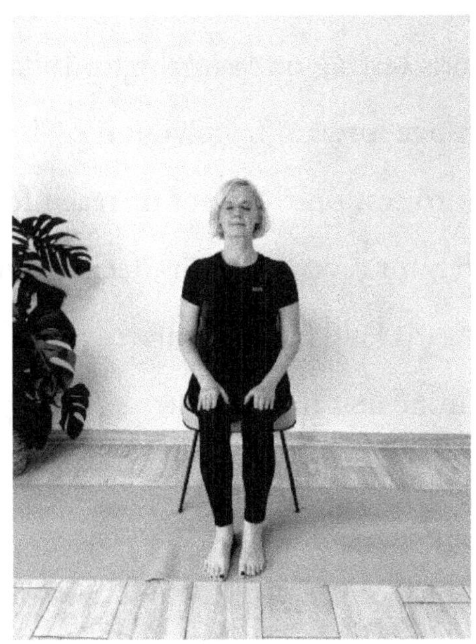
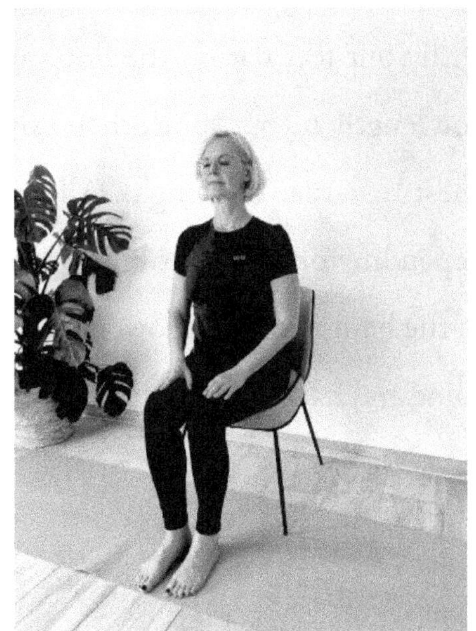

2. **Seated Cat-Cow Stretch:** Sit towards the front edge of your chair with your feet flat on the floor and your hands resting on your knees. Inhale as you arch your back and lift your chest towards the ceiling, coming into Cow Pose. Exhale as you round your spine and tuck your chin towards your chest, coming into Cat Pose. Flow smoothly between these two poses with your breath, moving with grace and ease. Seated Cat-Cow Stretch helps to mobilize the spine, increase flexibility, and build core strength.

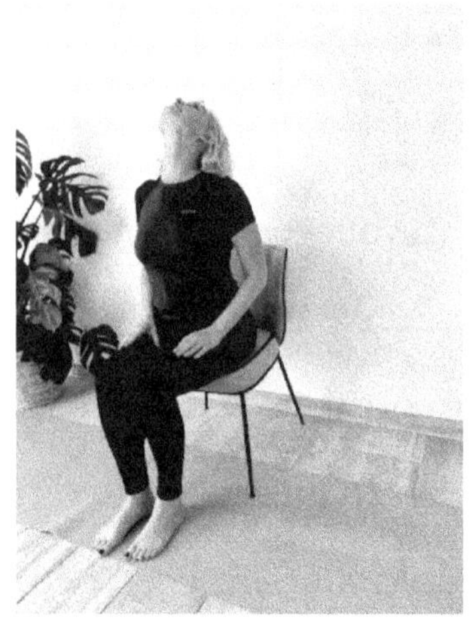 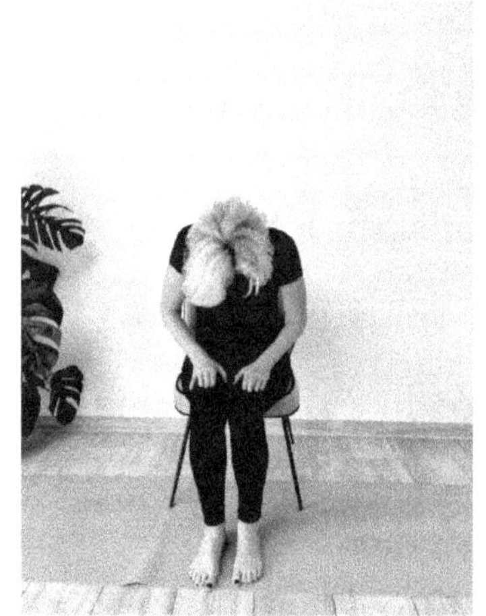 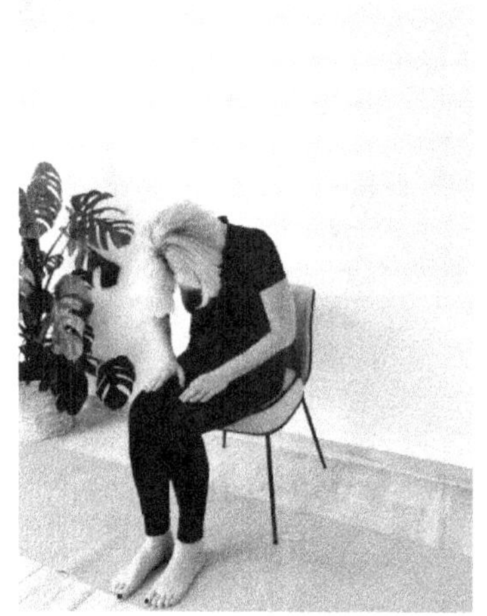

3. **Seated Forward Fold (Paschimottanasana):** Sit towards the front edge of your chair with your feet flat on the floor and your hands resting on your thighs. Inhale deeply as you lengthen your spine, then exhale as you hinge forward from your hips, bringing your chest towards your thighs. Allow your hands to rest on the floor or reach for your feet, depending on your flexibility. Hold the stretch for several breaths, feeling a deep release in the hamstrings and lower back. Seated Forward Fold helps to improve flexibility in the spine and hamstrings, while also calming the mind and reducing stress.

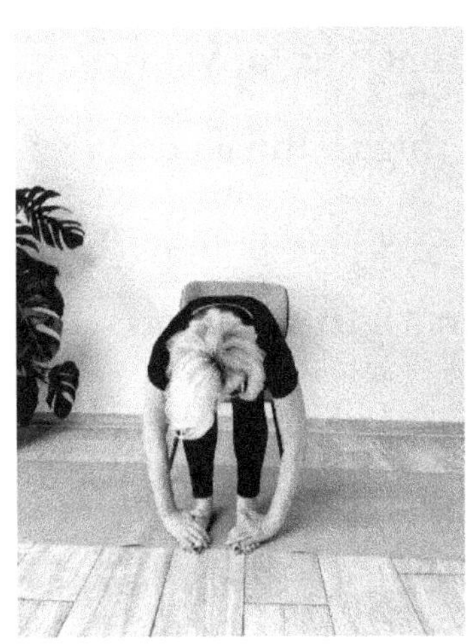 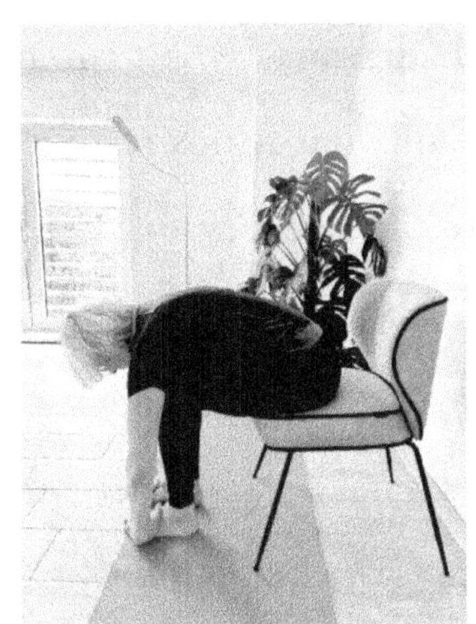 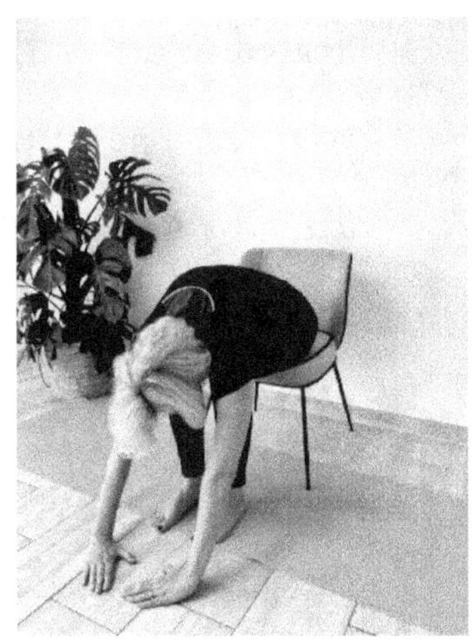

4.   **Seated Twist (Ardha Matsyendrasana):** Sit tall in your chair with your feet flat on the floor and your hands resting on your knees. Inhale deeply as you lengthen your spine, then exhale as you twist to the right, bringing your left hand to the outside of your right knee and your right hand behind you on the chair. Hold the twist for several breaths, feeling a gentle stretch in the spine and shoulders. Inhale to return to center, then exhale to repeat on the left side. Seated Twist helps to improve spinal mobility, stimulate digestion, and detoxify the body.

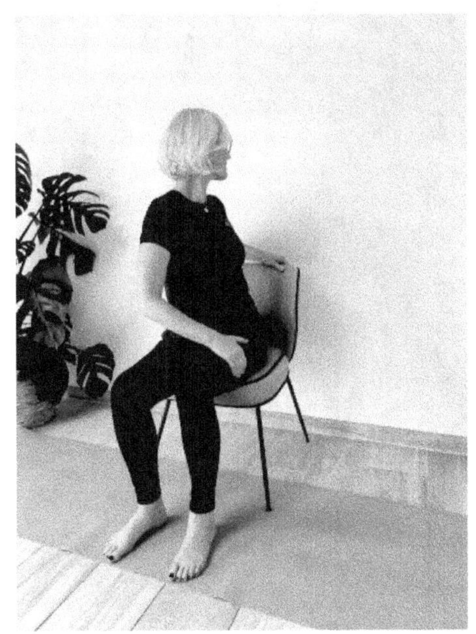 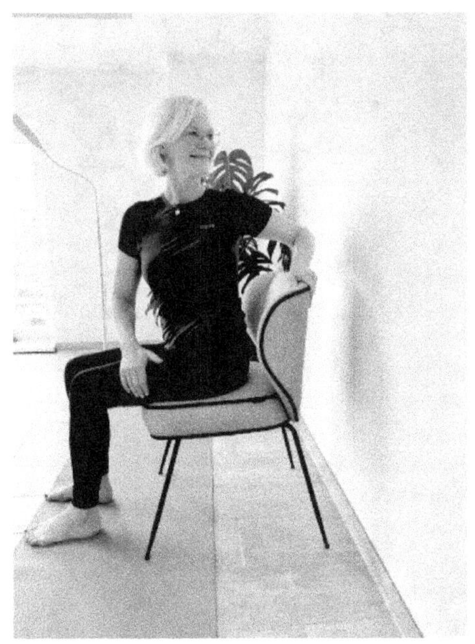

5. **Seated Warrior II (Virabhadrasana II):** Sit towards the front edge of your chair with your feet flat on the floor and your hands resting on your thighs. Inhale deeply as you extend your right leg out to the side, bending your right knee and aligning it with your ankle. Exhale as you extend your arms out to the sides, parallel to the floor, with your palms facing down. Gaze over your right fingertips, feeling strong and confident like a warrior. Hold the pose for several breaths, then inhale to return to center and repeat on the left side. Seated Warrior II helps to build strength in the legs, open the hips, and improve concentration and focus.

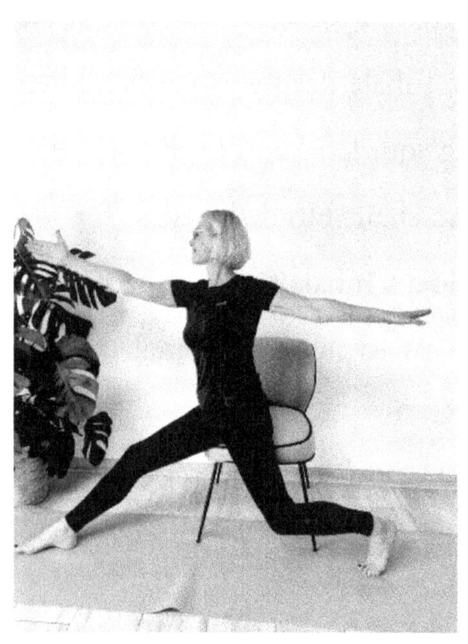 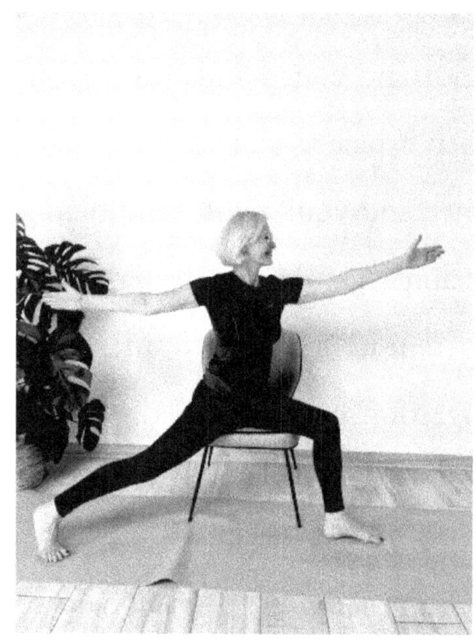

Day 2 - Day 9 – Day 16 – Day 23: Mobility Improvement

Improving mobility is crucial for maintaining independence and vitality, especially as we age. In this section, we'll delve deeper into exercises and techniques specifically designed to enhance mobility and flexibility, allowing you to move more freely and with greater ease in your daily activities.

Start your daily Yoga Routines with Breathwork and Warm-Up Exercises.

1. **Seated Spinal Twist with Extended Arm Reach:** Sit tall in your chair with your feet flat on the floor and your hands resting on your thighs. Inhale deeply as you lengthen your spine, then exhale as you twist to the right, placing your left hand on the outside of your right knee and reaching your right arm behind you. Hold the twist for a few breaths, feeling the stretch in your spine and shoulders. Inhale to return to center, then exhale to repeat on the left side. This exercise improves spinal mobility and stretches the muscles along the back and sides of the body.

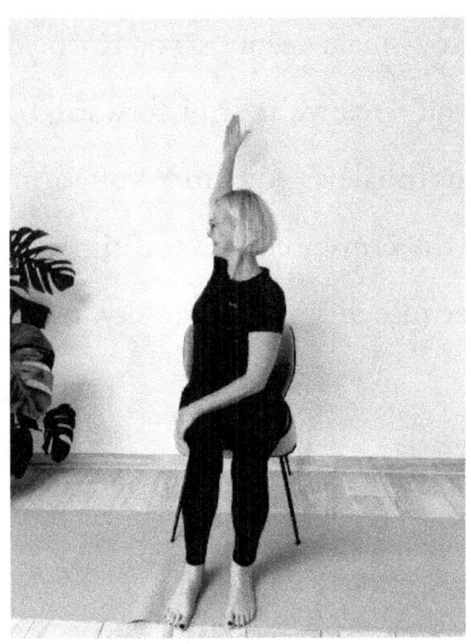
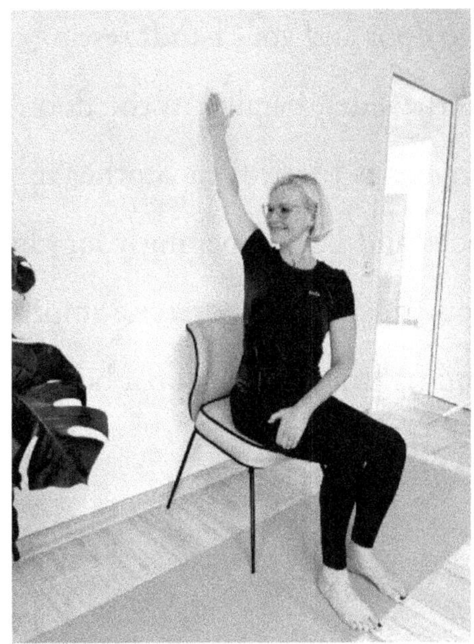

2. **Seated Hip Opener with Knee Lift:** Sit towards the front edge of your chair with your feet flat on the floor and your hands resting on your thighs. Inhale deeply as you lift your right knee towards your chest, clasping your hands around your knee if possible. Hold the knee lift for a few breaths, feeling the stretch in your hip flexors and quadriceps. Release and repeat on the left side. This exercise improves hip mobility and flexibility, helping to alleviate stiffness and discomfort.

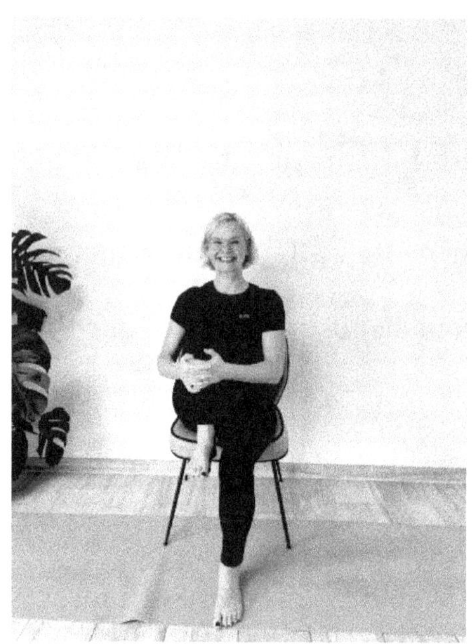

3. **Seated Shoulder Opener with Arm Circles:** Sit tall in your chair with your feet flat on the floor and your hands resting on your thighs. Inhale deeply as you reach your arms out to the sides, parallel to the floor. Exhale as you circle your arms forward, bringing your fingertips towards each other in front of you. Inhale as you circle your arms out to the sides and back, opening your chest. Repeat the arm circles several times, moving with your breath. This exercise improves shoulder mobility and flexibility, relieving tension and tightness in the upper body.

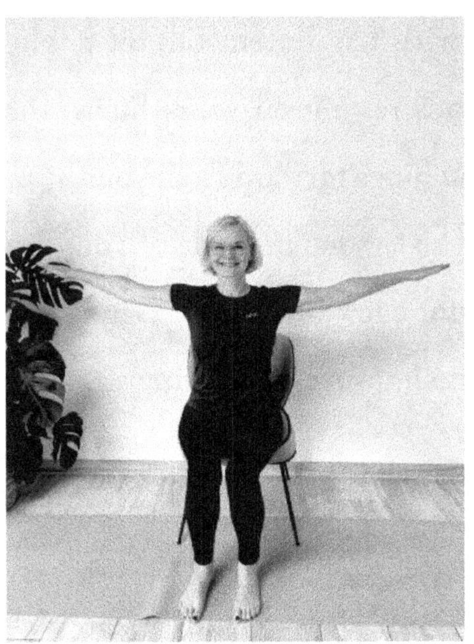

4. **Seated Side Stretch with Extended Arm Reach:** Sit towards the front edge of your chair with your feet flat on the floor and your hands resting on your thighs. Inhale deeply as you reach your right arm overhead, stretching towards the left side of the room. Exhale as you lean to the left, feeling the stretch along the right side of your body. Hold the side stretch for a few breaths, then inhale to return to center and repeat on the opposite side. This exercise improves lateral mobility and stretches the muscles along the sides of the body.

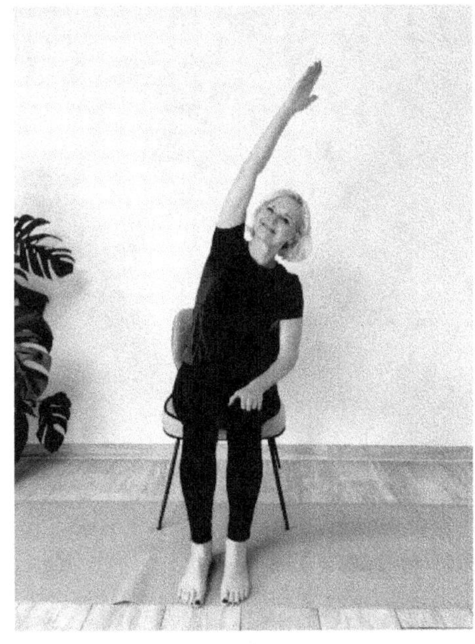
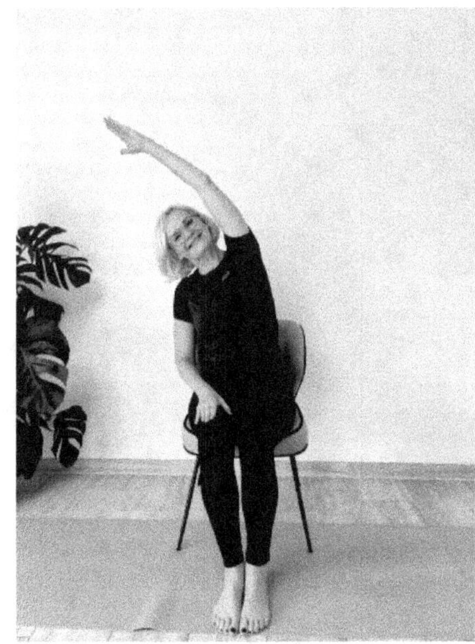

5. **Seated Forward Fold with Leg Extension:** Sit tall in your chair with your feet flat on the floor and your hands resting on your thighs. Inhale deeply as you lengthen your spine, then exhale as you hinge forward from your hips, bringing your chest towards your thighs. Extend your right leg out in front of you, flexing your foot towards your face. Hold the forward fold for a few breaths, then inhale to return to center and repeat with the left leg. This exercise improves hamstring flexibility and stretches the muscles along the back of the legs.

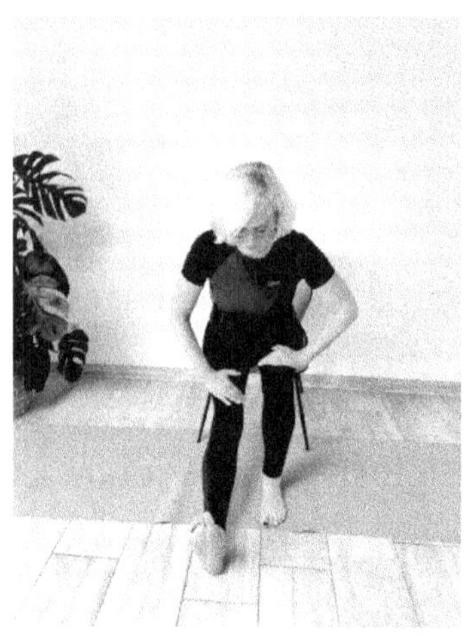 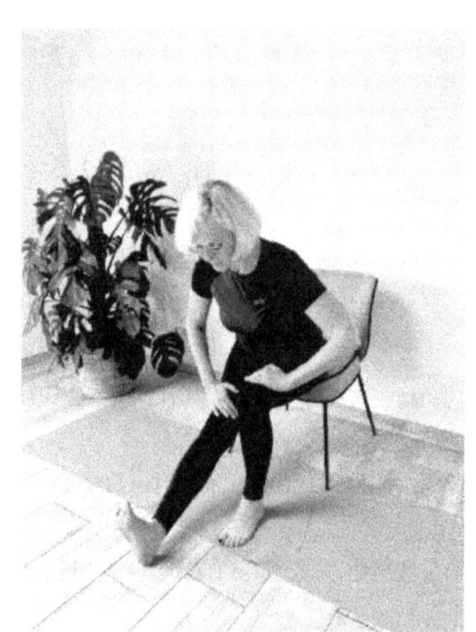 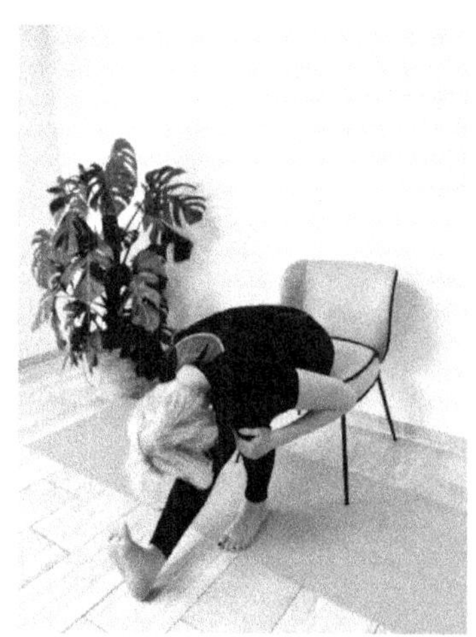

Day 3 – Day 10 – Day 17 – Day 24: Poses for Heart Health

Incorporate these Chair Yoga poses into your daily routine to support heart health, improve circulation, and enhance overall well-being. Remember to move with awareness and listen to your body's cues, modifying the poses as needed to suit your individual needs and abilities.

Start your daily Yoga Routines with Breathwork and Warm-Up Exercises.

1. **Seated Heart Opener:** Sit comfortably in your chair with your feet flat on the floor and your hands resting on your thighs. Inhale deeply as you lengthen your spine, then exhale as you gently arch your upper back and lift your chest towards the ceiling. Keep your shoulders relaxed and your chin parallel to the floor. Hold the pose for a few breaths, feeling a gentle stretch across the front of your chest. This pose opens the heart center, improves circulation, and promotes emotional well-being.

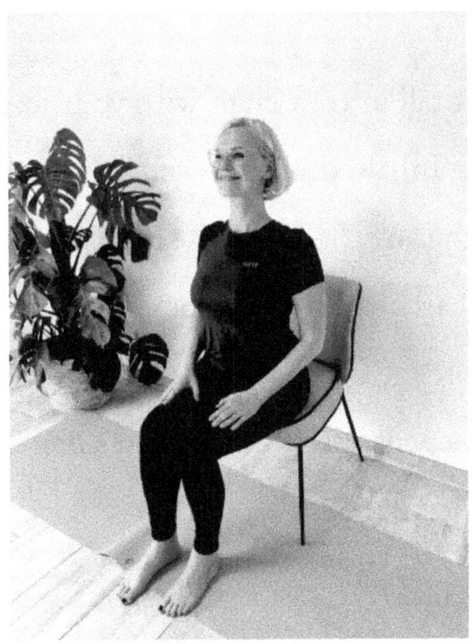

2. **Seated Forward Fold with Chest Expansion:** Sit towards the front edge of your chair with your feet flat on the floor and your hands resting on your thighs. Inhale deeply as you lengthen your spine, then exhale as you hinge forward from your hips, bringing your chest towards your thighs. Interlace your fingers behind your back and gently straighten your arms, lifting them towards the ceiling. Hold the forward fold with chest expansion for a few breaths, feeling a deep stretch in your chest and shoulders. This pose improves circulation to the heart and lungs, while also relieving tension in the upper body.

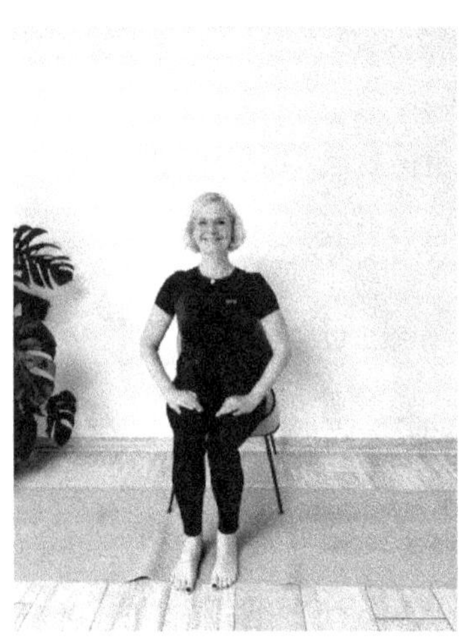 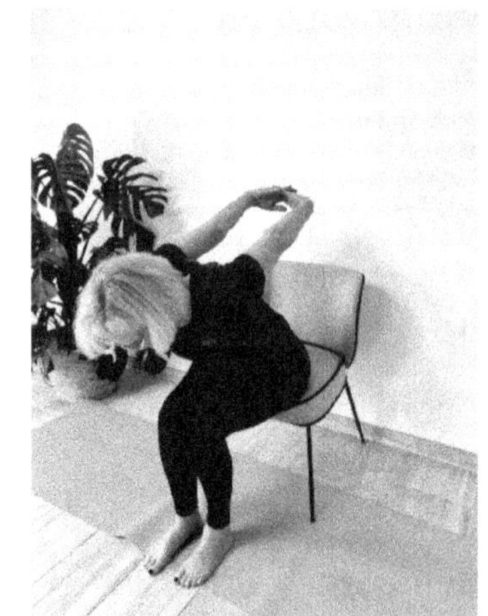 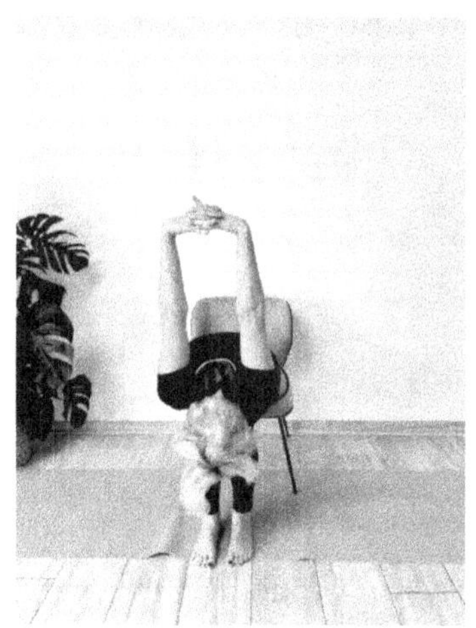

3. **Seated Camel Pose:** Sit tall in your chair with your feet flat on the floor and your hands resting on your thighs. Inhale deeply as you lengthen your spine, then exhale as you slowly lean back, bringing your hands to the back of the chair for support. Lift your chest towards the ceiling and arch your upper back, feeling a gentle stretch across the front of your body. Hold the pose for a few breaths, then inhale to return to an upright position. Seated Camel Pose opens the chest and increases lung capacity, promoting cardiovascular health and vitality.

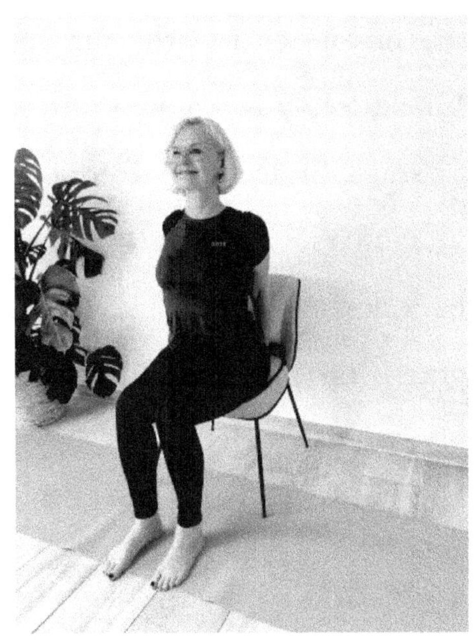 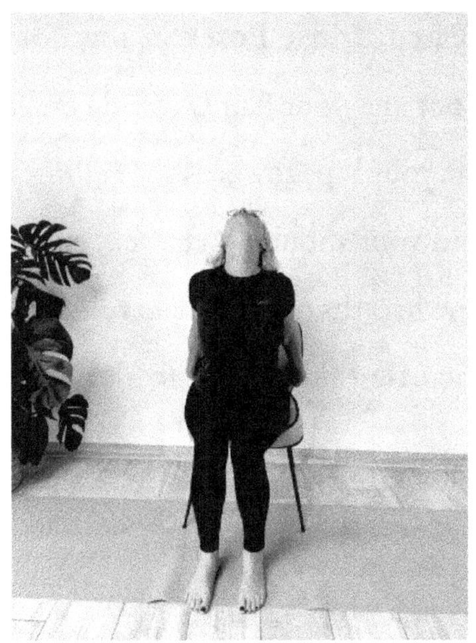

4. **Seated Twist with Heart Mudra:** Sit tall in your chair with your feet flat on the floor and your hands resting on your thighs. Inhale deeply as you lengthen your spine, then exhale as you twist to the right, bringing your left hand to the outside of your right knee and your right hand to your heart center. Press your palms together in prayer position, creating a heart mudra with your hands. Hold the twist for a few breaths, then inhale to return to center and repeat on the left side. Seated Twist with Heart Mudra improves circulation and opens the heart center, fostering a sense of love and compassion.

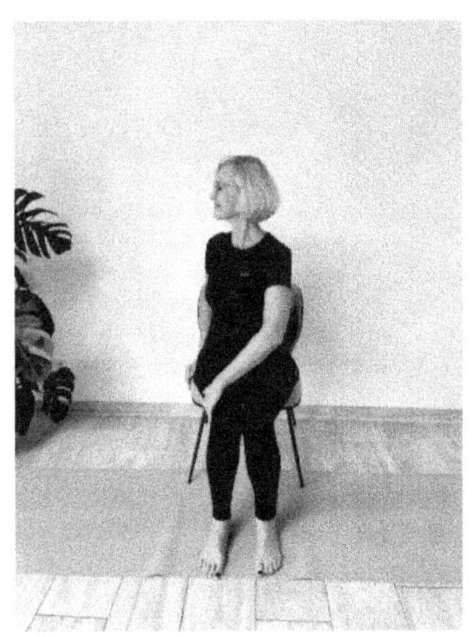 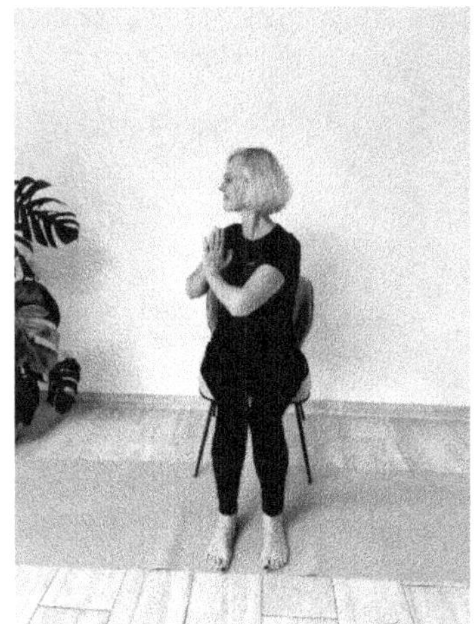 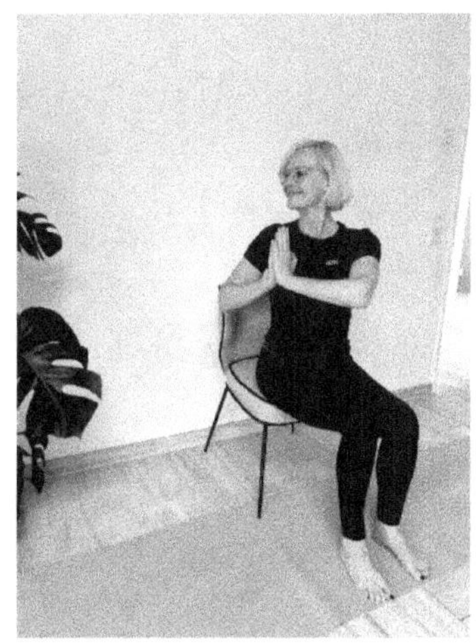

5. **Seated Bridge Pose:** Sit towards the front edge of your chair with your feet flat on the floor and your hands resting on your thighs. Inhale deeply as you press into your feet and lift your hips towards the ceiling, coming into a seated bridge pose. Keep your chest lifted and your shoulders relaxed, engaging your core muscles for stability. Hold the pose for a few breaths, then exhale to lower your hips back down to the chair. Seated Bridge Pose increases blood flow to the heart and strengthens the muscles of the chest and upper back.

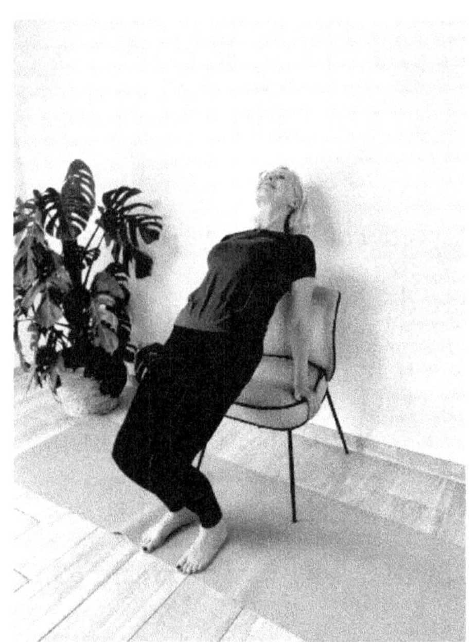 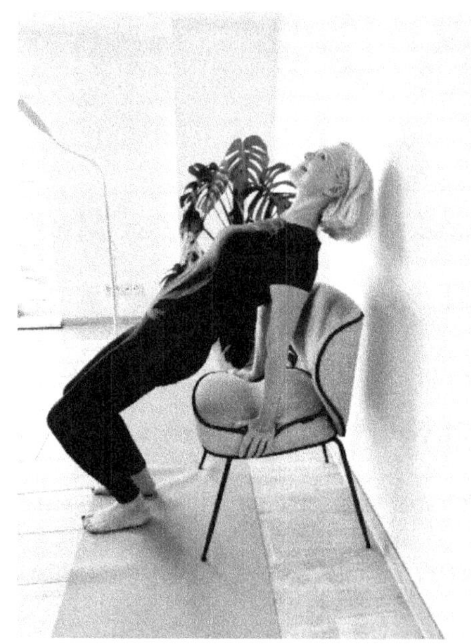

Day 4 – Day 11 – Day 18 – Day 25: Building Strength

Incorporate these Chair Yoga exercises into your routine to build strength, improve muscle tone, and enhance overall physical fitness. Remember to move with intention and listen to your body, modifying the exercises as needed to suit your individual needs and abilities.

Start your daily Yoga Routines with Breathwork and Warm-Up Exercises.

1. **Seated Warrior III:** Sit tall in your chair with your feet flat on the floor and your hands resting on your thighs. Inhale deeply as you engage your core muscles and lift your right leg off the floor, extending it straight behind you. Keep your hips squared and your toes pointing towards the ground. Reach your arms forward, parallel to the floor, with your palms facing each other. Hold the pose for a few breaths, feeling the strength and stability in your standing leg and core. Repeat on the other side. Seated Warrior III strengthens the legs, core, and stabilizing muscles, improving balance and coordination.

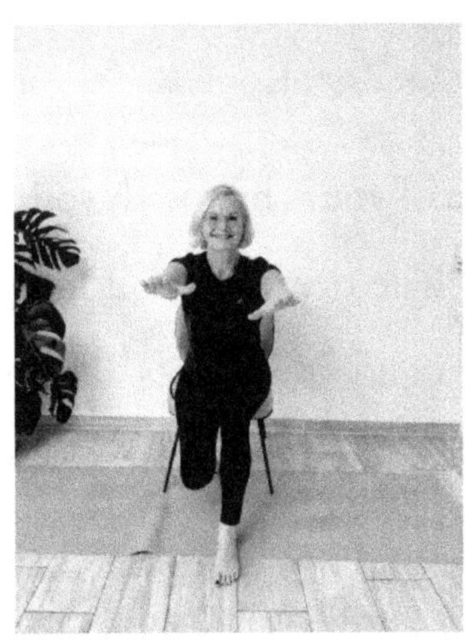
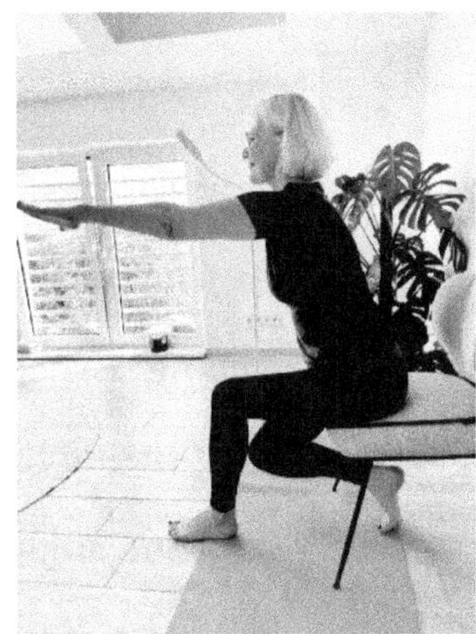
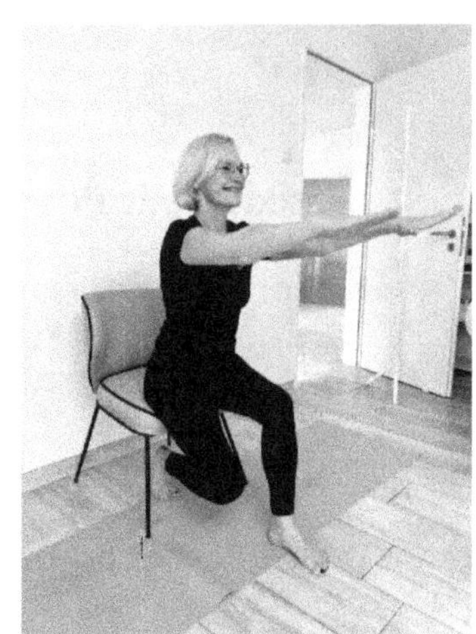

2. **Seated Boat Pose:** Sit towards the front edge of your chair with your feet flat on the floor and your hands resting on your thighs. Inhale deeply as you lift your feet off the floor, bringing your knees towards your chest. Extend your arms forward, parallel to the floor, with your palms facing each other. Engage your core muscles and straighten your legs, forming a V-shape with your body. Hold the pose for a few breaths, feeling the strength and activation in your core. Seated Boat Pose strengthens the abdominal muscles, hip flexors, and lower back, improving core stability and posture.

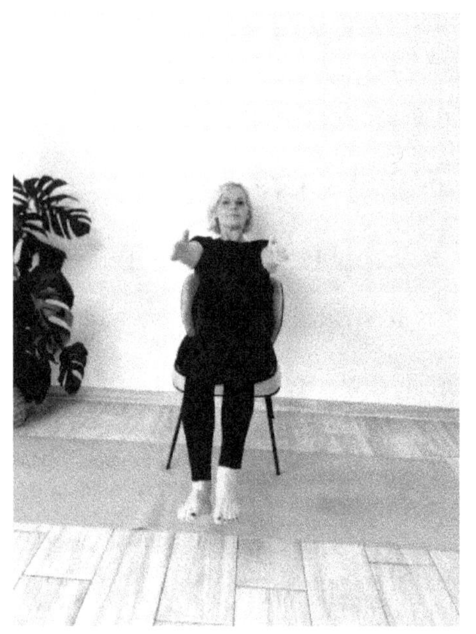 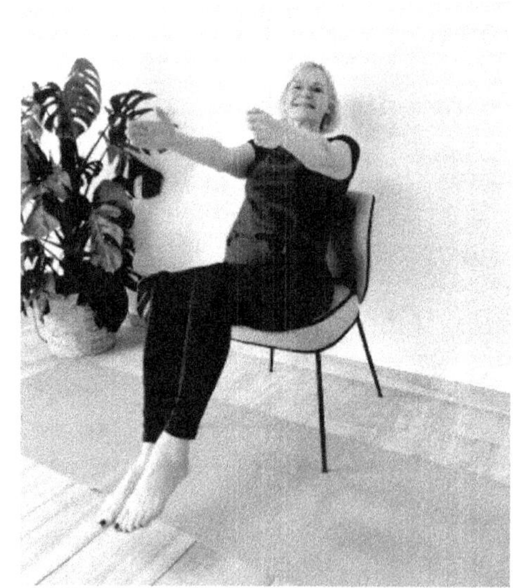

3. **Seated Chair Pose (Utkatasana):** Sit towards the front edge of your chair with your feet flat on the floor and your hands resting on your thighs. Inhale deeply as you lift your arms overhead, reaching towards the ceiling. Exhale as you bend your knees and lower your hips towards the floor, as if you were sitting back into a chair. Keep your weight in your heels and your knees stacked over your ankles. Hold the pose for a few breaths, feeling the strength and activation in your quadriceps and glutes. Seated Chair Pose builds strength in the lower body and improves stability and urance.

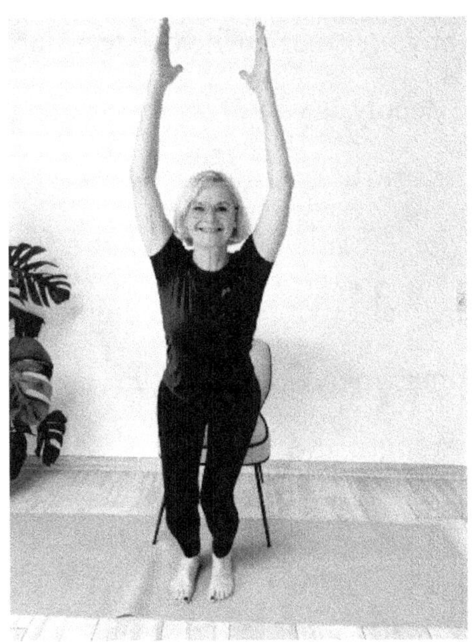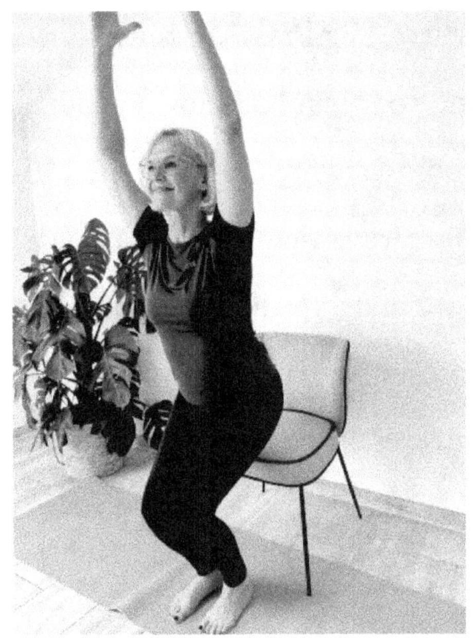

4. **Seated Push-Ups:** Sit towards the front edge of your chair with your hands gripping the sides of the seat, fingers facing forward. Inhale deeply as you bend your elbows and lower your chest towards the chair, keeping your back straight and your elbows close to your body. Exhale as you push through your palms and straighten your arms, lifting your chest back up to the starting position. Repeat for several repetitions, moving with control and focusing on engaging your chest, shoulders, and triceps. Seated Push-Ups build upper body strength and improve functional fitness.

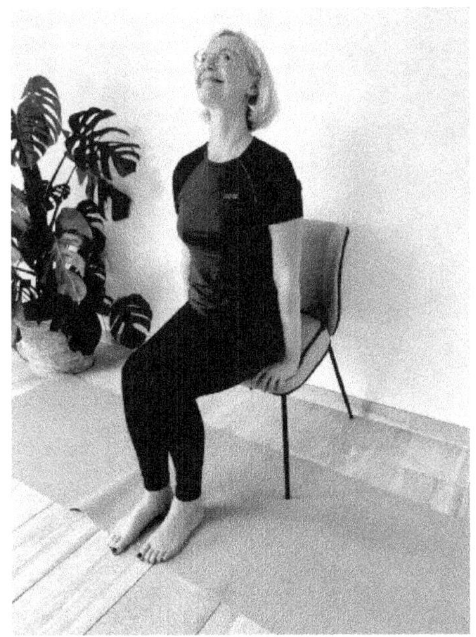

5. **Seated Leg Press:** Sit towards the front edge of your chair with your feet flat on the floor and your hands resting on your thighs. Inhale deeply as you press your right foot into the floor, straightening your right leg and lifting it off the ground. Exhale as you release and lower your right foot back down. Repeat on the left side, pressing your left foot into the floor and straightening your left leg. Continue to alternate legs, moving with control and focusing on engaging your quadriceps and hamstrings. Seated Leg Press strengthens the muscles of the legs and improves lower body strength and stability.

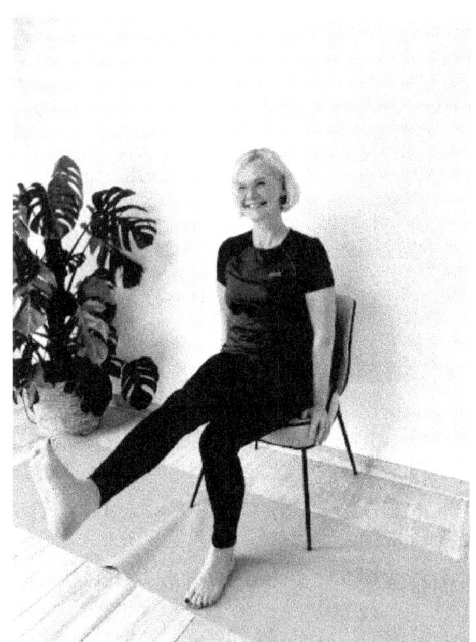

Day 5 – Day 12 – Day 19 – Day 26: Improved Posture and Alignment

Incorporate these Chair Yoga exercises into your daily routine to improve posture, alignment, and overall spinal health. Remember to move with mindfulness and listen to your body's cues, modifying the exercises as needed to suit your individual needs and abilities.

Start your daily Yoga Routines with Breathwork and Warm-Up Exercises.

1. **Seated Shoulder Rolls:** Sit tall in your chair with your feet flat on the floor and your hands resting on your thighs. Inhale deeply as you shrug your shoulders up towards your ears. Exhale as you roll your shoulders back and down, drawing your shoulder blades towards each other. Repeat this movement, rolling your shoulders in circles, alternating between forward and backward rolls. Focus on relaxing the muscles of the neck and shoulders and maintaining proper alignment throughout the movement. Seated Shoulder Rolls relieve tension in the upper back and neck, improving posture and alignment.

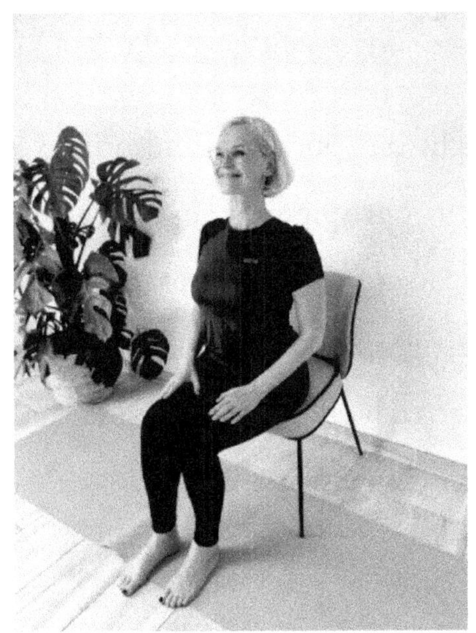
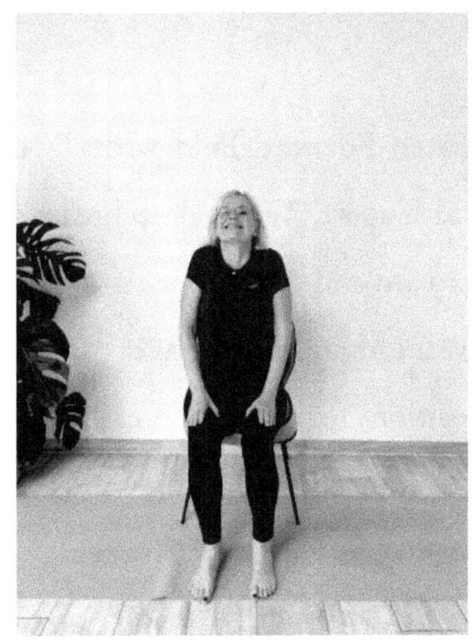

2. **Seated Side Stretch:** Sit towards the front edge of your chair with your feet flat on the floor and your hands resting on your thighs. Inhale deeply as you reach your right arm overhead, lengthening through the right side of your body. Exhale as you gently lean to the left, stretching your right arm towards the left side of the room. Keep both hips grounded on the chair and both feet flat on the floor. Hold the stretch for a few breaths, then inhale to return to an upright position and repeat on the other side. Seated Side Stretch opens the side body, improves spinal alignment, and relieves tension in the back and shoulders.

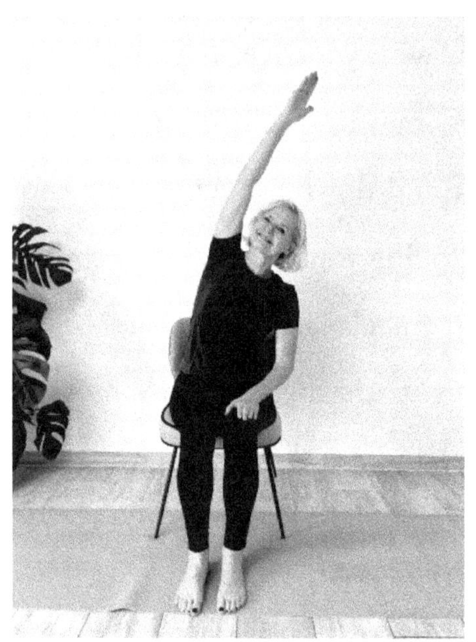 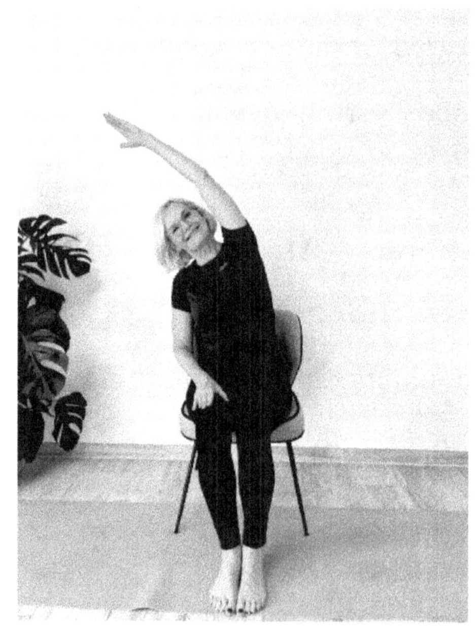

3. **Seated Forward Fold with Twist:** Sit upright on your chair and bring your feet hip-width apart. Take a deep breath and lengthen your spine. Then, with a flat back, hinge forward and reach your right hand to the outside of your left foot. Extend your left arm overhead and gently twist your torso to the right, lifting your gaze upward. Hold the position for several breaths, feeling the stretch along your spine and your side abdominals. Inhale deeply and return to center before switching sides.

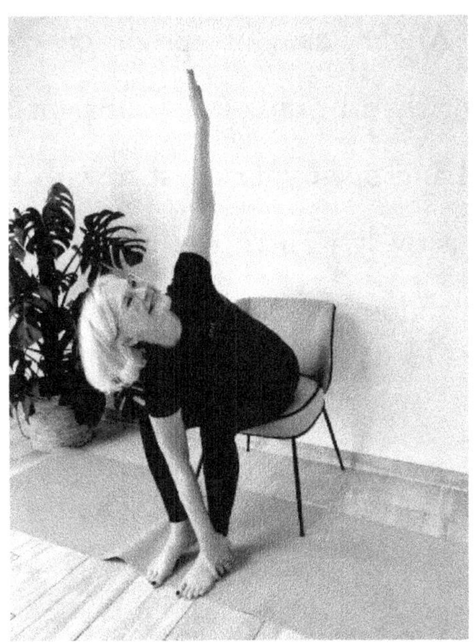

4. **Seated Half Moon Pose:** Sit upright on your chair and ground your feet firmly on the floor. Lift your right arm overhead and clasp your left wrist. Then, slowly lean to the right, bringing your left arm overhead and stretching your left side. Hold the position for several breaths as you actively lean to the left and lengthen your right side. Feel the stretch along your side abdominals and ribs. Inhale deeply and return to center before switching sides.

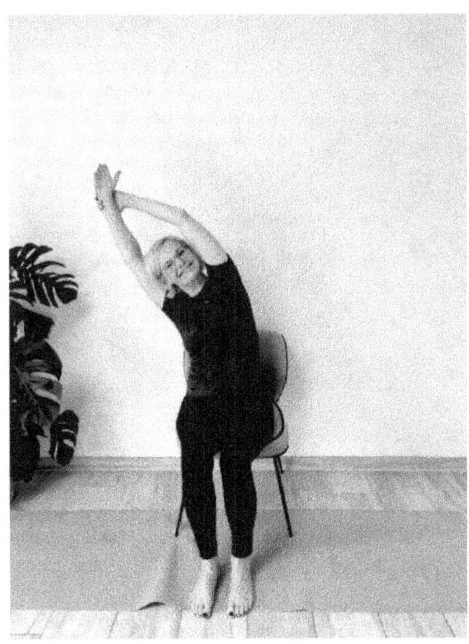

5. **Seated Extended Side Angle Pose:** Sit upright on your chair and bring your feet hip-width apart. Bend your right arm and place your right elbow on your right thigh. Extend your left arm overhead and open your chest toward the ceiling. Hold the position for several breaths as you actively lean to the right and lengthen your left side. Feel the stretch along your side abdominals and ribs. Inhale deeply and return to center before switching sides.

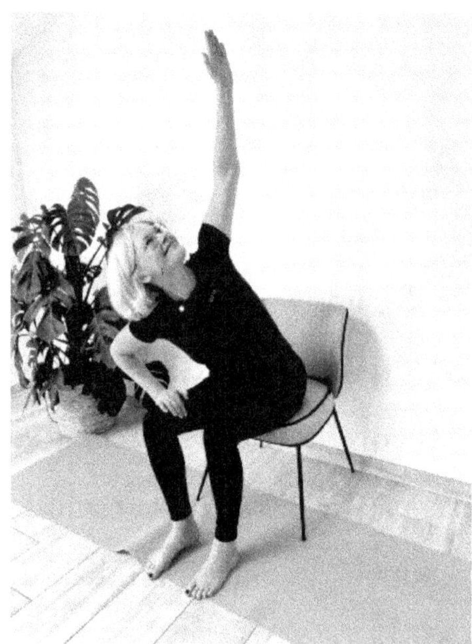

Day 6 – Day 13 – Day 20 – Day 27: Mobility and Strength Deepening

These advanced Chair Yoga exercises will help deepen mobility and strength, but remember to listen to your body and modify as needed. Enjoy the journey of exploration and growth in your practice!

Start your daily Yoga Routines with Breathwork and Warm-Up Exercises.

1. **Seated Crescent Moon:** Sit upright on your chair with feet flat on the floor. Inhale, then exhale as you reach your right arm up and over your head, creating a gentle stretch along your side body. Keep your left hand grounded on the chair seat for support. Hold for a few breaths, feeling the stretch, then switch sides.

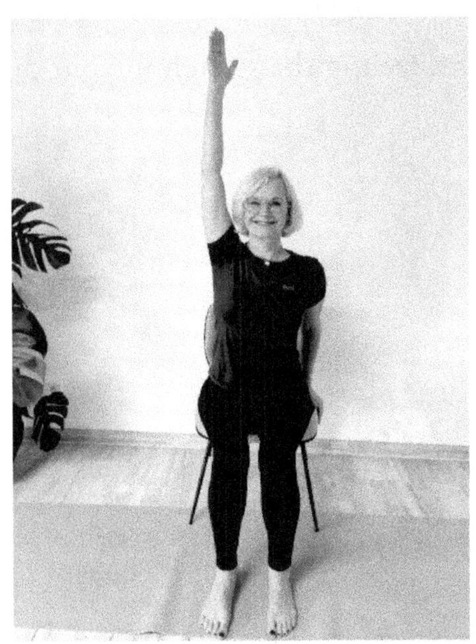 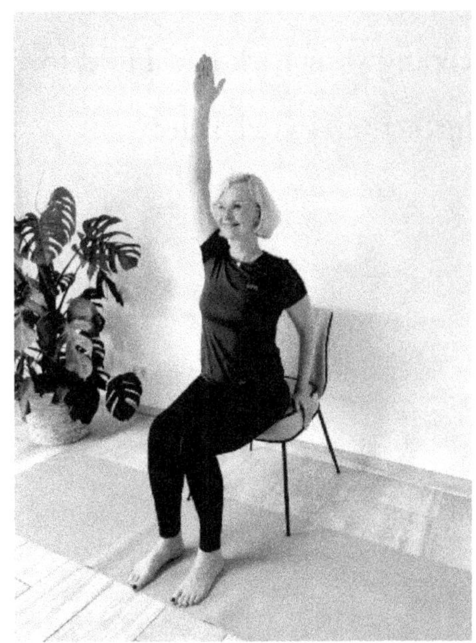

2. **Seated Warrior II:** Start seated with feet hip-width apart. Inhale and extend your arms out to the sides, palms facing down. Exhale and turn your torso to the right, bending your right knee and aligning it over your ankle. Keep your left leg extended and foot firmly planted. Hold the pose for a few breaths, feeling the strength in your legs and core, then switch sides.

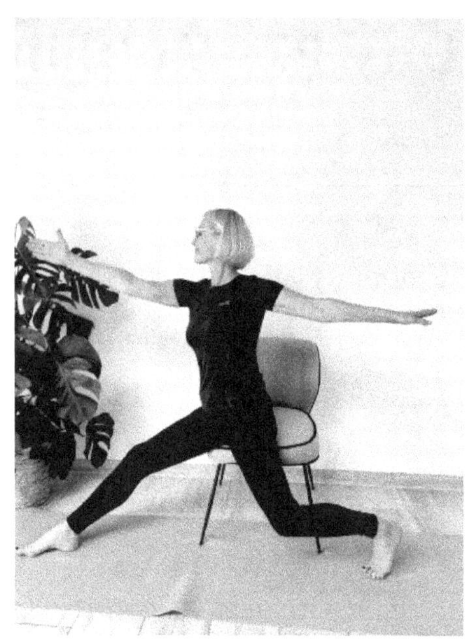 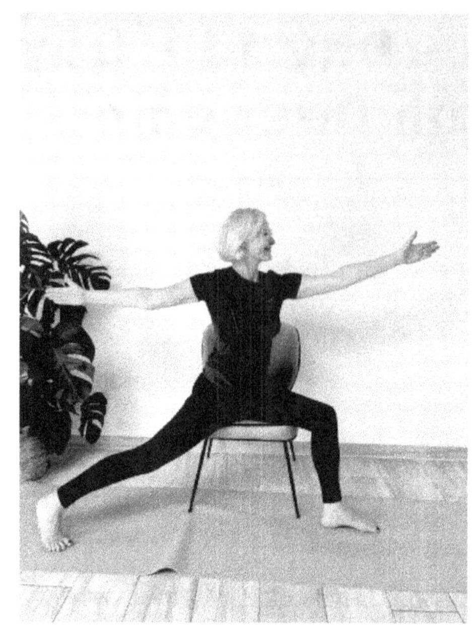

3. **Seated Pigeon Pose:** Sit upright on your chair and cross your right ankle over your left knee, creating a figure-four shape with your legs. Flex your right foot to protect your knee. Inhale, lengthen your spine, and exhale as you hinge forward from your hips, keeping your back flat. Hold for a few breaths, feeling the stretch in your outer hip and glutes, then switch sides.

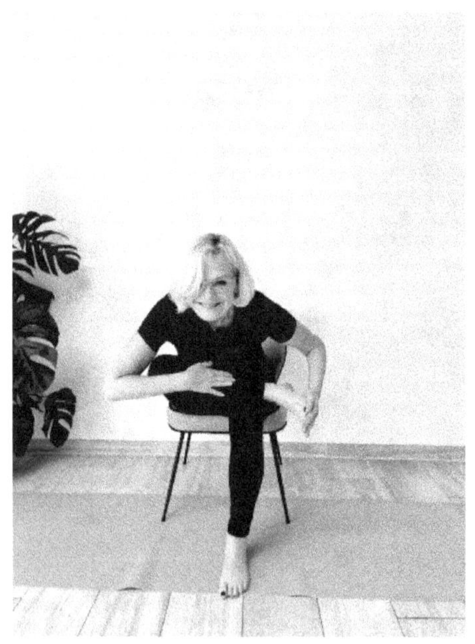 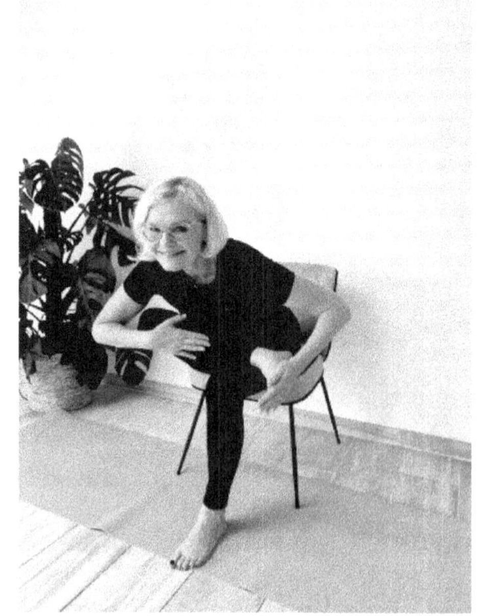

4. **Seated Boat Pose:** Sit towards the front edge of your chair with knees bent and feet flat on the floor. Hold onto the sides of the chair for support. Inhale, lengthen your spine, and exhale as you lift your feet off the floor, bringing your shins parallel to the ground. Engage your core and hold for a few breaths, feeling the strength in your abdominals, then release back down.

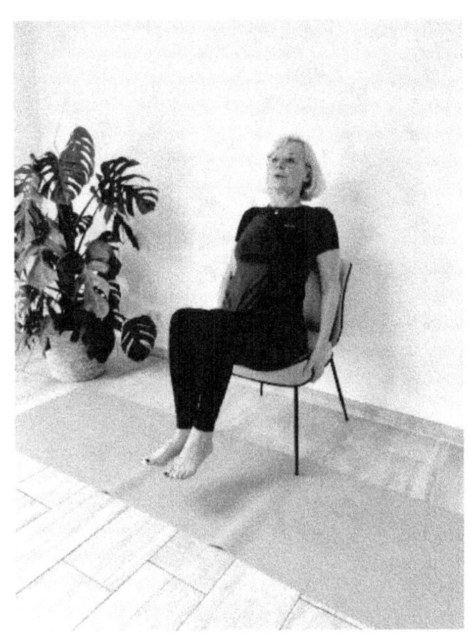
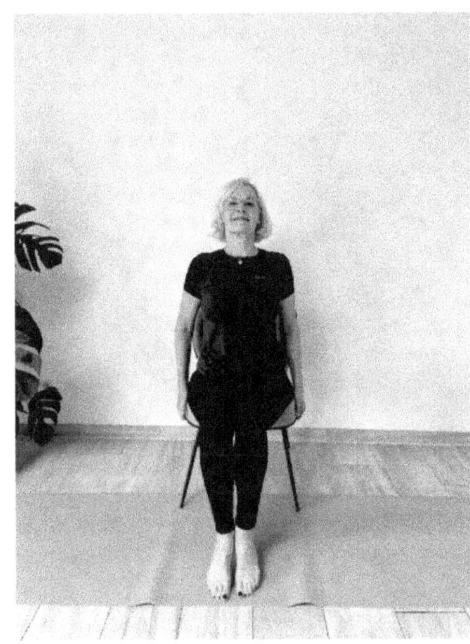

5. **Seated Plank Pose:** Sit upright on your chair with hands placed on the seat beside your hips, fingers pointing forward. Inhale, engage your core, and lift your hips off the chair, coming into a seated plank position. Keep your body in a straight line from head to heels, and hold for a few breaths, feeling the strength in your arms, core, and legs. Release back down with control.

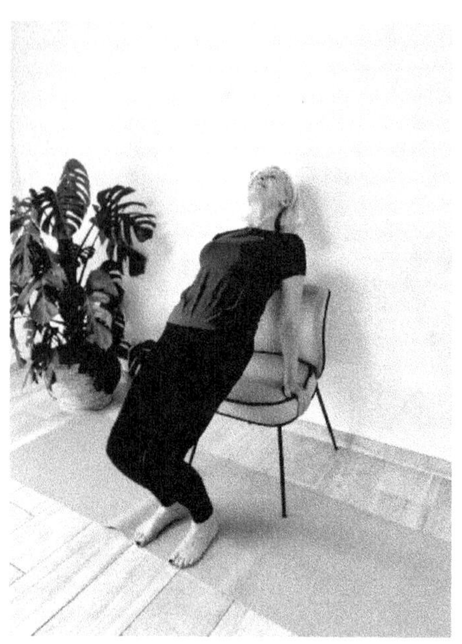 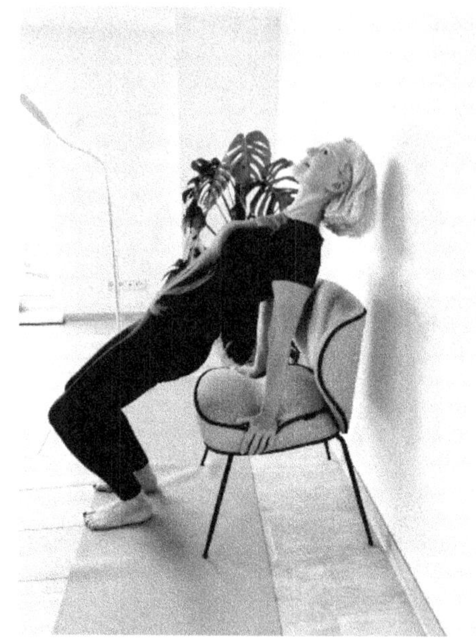

Day 7 – Day 14 – Day 21 – Day 28: Stress Reduction and Relaxation

These Chair Yoga exercises for stress reduction and relaxation will help you unwind and find calmness in your body and mind. Practice them regularly to cultivate a sense of inner peace and well-being.

Start your daily Yoga Routines with Breathwork and Warm-Up Exercises.

1. **Seated Forward Fold with Gentle Neck Stretch:** Sit comfortably on your chair with feet flat on the floor. Inhale, then exhale as you hinge forward from your hips, bringing your chest towards your thighs. Allow your arms to hang loosely or rest them on your legs. Relax your neck and let your head hang heavy. Take deep breaths, feeling the release of tension in your back and neck.

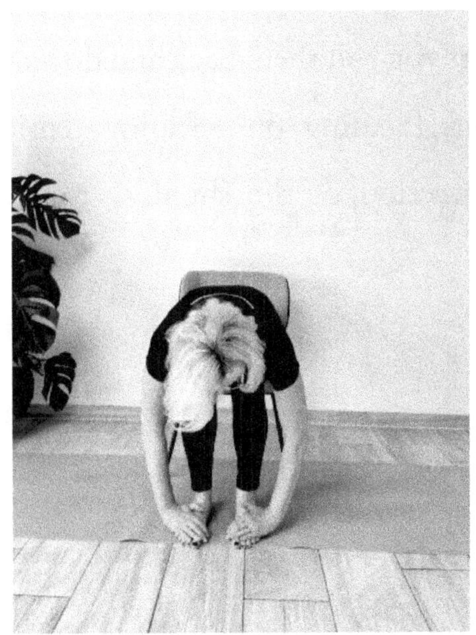
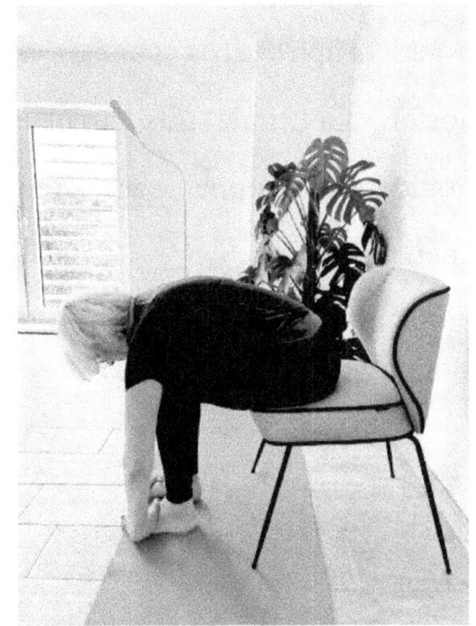

2. **Seated Cat-Cow Stretch:** Sit upright on your chair with hands resting on your knees. Inhale as you arch your back and lift your chest, allowing your belly to come forward (Cow Pose). Exhale as you round your spine, tucking your chin to your chest and drawing your belly button towards your spine (Cat Pose). Flow between these two poses with your breath, moving gently and rhythmically.

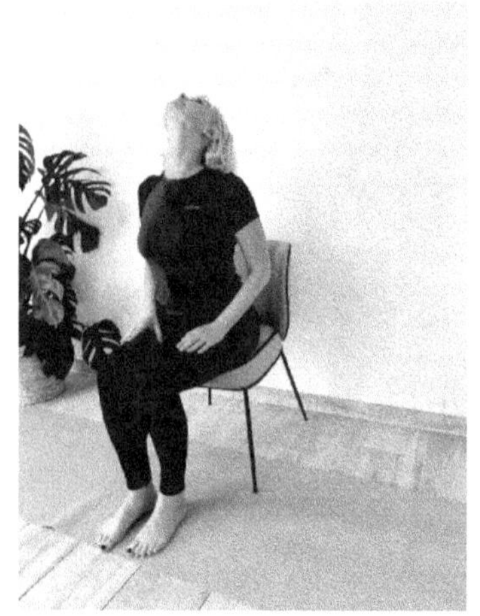
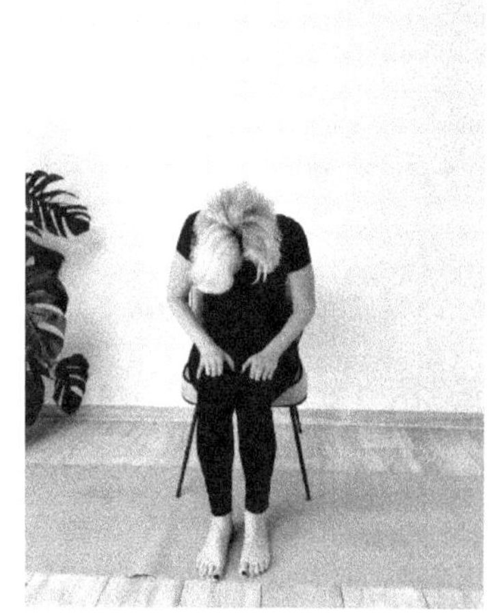
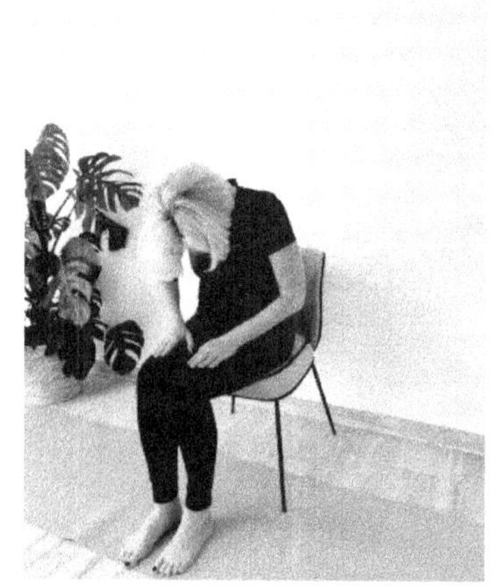

3. **Seated Shoulder Rolls:** Sit comfortably with feet flat on the floor. Inhale as you lift your shoulders up towards your ears, then exhale as you roll them back and down in a smooth motion. Continue this circular movement, focusing on releasing tension in your shoulders and upper back. Reverse the direction of the shoulder rolls after a few repetitions.

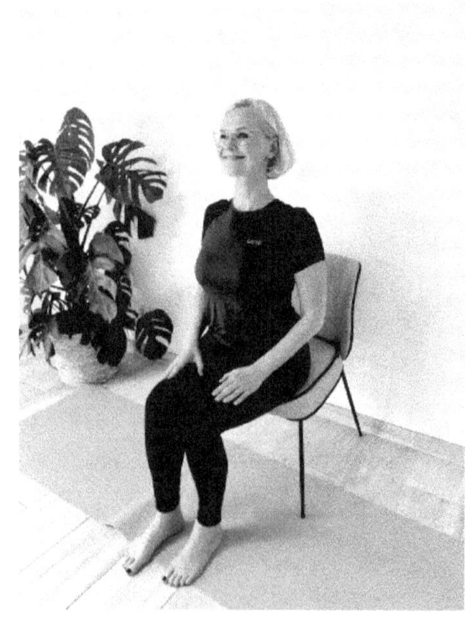
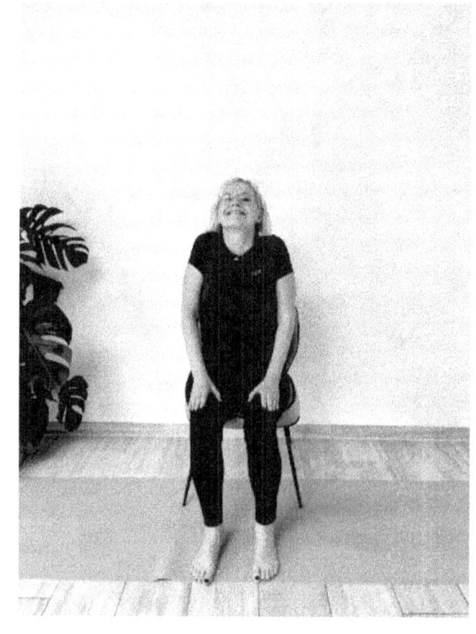

4. **Seated Twist and Release:** Sit tall on your chair with feet planted firmly on the ground. Inhale to lengthen your spine, and then exhale as you twist your torso to the right, placing your left hand on the outside of your right thigh and your right hand on the back of the chair. Hold the twist for a few breaths, and then inhale to return to center and repeat on the other side. Feel the gentle release of tension in your spine with each twist.

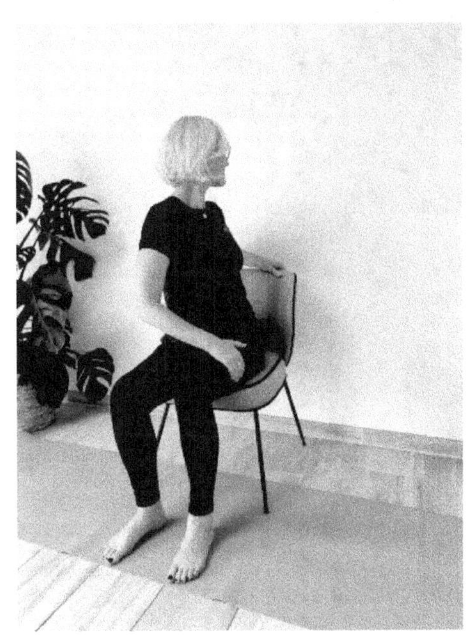 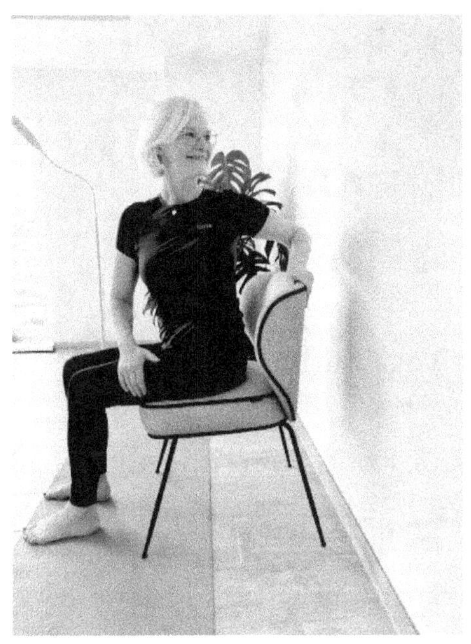

5. **Seated Guided Meditation:** Sit comfortably with your back supported by the chair and your feet flat on the floor. Close your eyes and take several deep breaths to settle into the present moment. Begin to focus on your breath, observing the inhale and exhale without judgment. Allow your body to relax with each breath, letting go of any tension or stress. Stay in this meditative state for a few minutes, enjoying the peace and tranquility it brings.

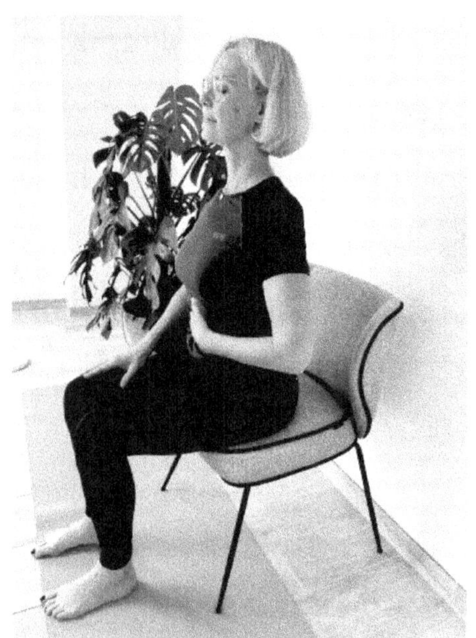 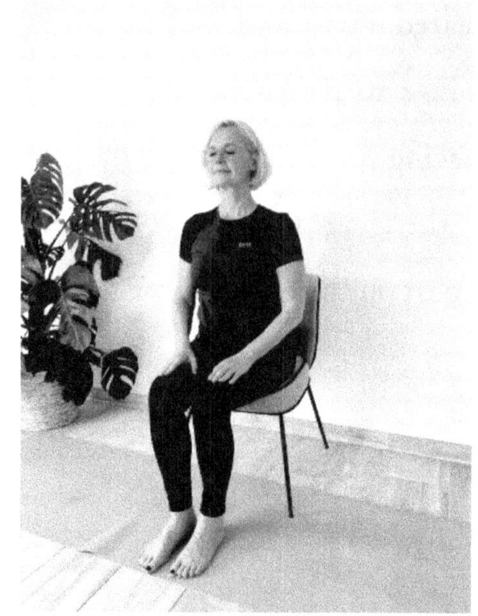

Dear Chair Yoga Enthusiast,

Congratulations on completing the Chair Yoga challenge for seniors over 60! I'm absolutely thrilled and grateful that you chose my book to guide you on this journey. It takes courage to embark on something new, and I admire your willingness to take that leap.

As you wrap up this challenge, I want to encourage you to keep going. Don't ever stop exploring and evolving in your practice. Each time you step onto your yoga mat, you're not just stretching your body, but also expanding your mind and nurturing your spirit.

Remember, it's not about perfection—it's about progress. Whether you're mastering a difficult pose or simply finding stillness in your breath, every moment on the mat is an opportunity for growth.

Thank you for allowing me to be a part of your yoga journey. I hope this book has brought you joy, peace, and a deeper connection to yourself. Keep shining brightly, my friend, and may your path be filled with love, laughter, and endless possibilities.

PART 7

CHAKRAS GUIDE

Dear Chair Yoga Enthusiast,

Welcome to the world of chakras! As we embark on this journey together, I am thrilled to guide you through the fascinating and transformative landscape of the seven energy centers that govern our physical, emotional, and spiritual well-being. With years of experience in the realm of Chair Yoga and a deep understanding of the challenges faced by those over 60, I am excited to share with you the wisdom and insights that have enriched my own life.

In this guide, we will delve into the ancient wisdom of chakras, exploring their significance and the profound impact they have on our lives. From the foundational understanding of what chakras are to practical techniques for balancing and harmonizing them, we will uncover the secrets to unlocking your fullest potential and experiencing greater harmony, vitality, and joy.

Through humor, empathy, and a touch of wisdom gained from my journey, I aim to make this exploration enlightening and enjoyable for you. So, let us embark on this adventure together, with open hearts and minds, as we discover the power and beauty of the chakra system.

What Are Chakras?

Chakras are the energy centers of the body, each corresponding to specific physical, emotional, and spiritual aspects of our being. The word "chakra" is derived from Sanskrit, meaning "wheel" or "disk," symbolizing the swirling vortex of energy within each center.

According to ancient Indian spiritual traditions, the human body contains seven main chakras, which align vertically from the base of the spine to the crown of the head. These chakras are believed to be interconnected, spinning wheels of energy that regulate the flow of prana, or life force, throughout the body.

Each chakra is associated with a specific color, element, mantra, and aspect of consciousness, representing different stages of our spiritual evolution. When the chakras are balanced and aligned, energy flows freely, promoting physical health, emotional well-being, and spiritual growth. However, imbalances or blockages in the chakras can lead to various physical ailments, emotional disturbances, and spiritual disconnection.

Understanding and working with the chakras can help us cultivate greater awareness, healing, and transformation in our lives. By harmonizing the flow of energy within the chakras, we can achieve a state of balance, vitality, and inner harmony.

How Many Chakras Are There in the Body?

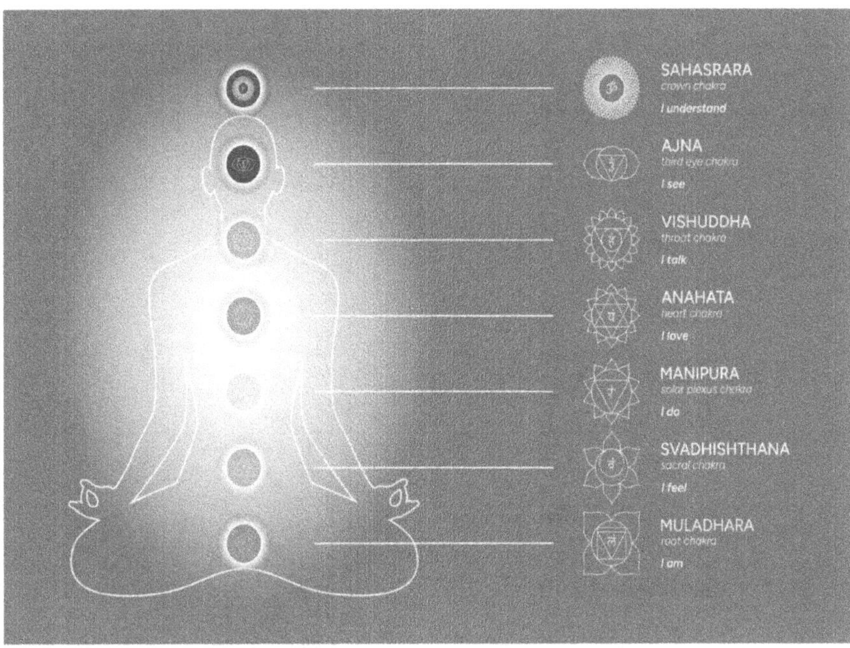

While there are numerous energy centers in the body, traditional teachings focus on seven main chakras:

- Muladhara Chakra - Root Chakra

- Svadhishthana Chakra – Sacral Chakra

- Manipura Chakra – Solar Plexus Chakra

- Anahata Chakra – Heart Chakra

- Vishuddha Chakra – Throat Chakra

- Ajna Chakra – Third Eye Chakra

- Sahastrara Chakra – Crown Chakra

Does a Chakra have a Shape?

Although chakras are often depicted as swirling vortexes or discs of energy, they do not have a fixed physical form. Rather, they are energetic centers that regulate the flow of prana or life force throughout the body. However, envisioning chakras as wheels or discs helps to visualize their concept and understand their function better.

How do Chakras Work?

Chakras work through the flow of energy passing through them, influencing various aspects of our physical, emotional, and spiritual well-being. When the chakras are balanced and active, we can experience a sense of harmony, vitality, and inner peace. They are important because they help us balance our energy, release blockages, and attain higher consciousness. By working with the chakras, we can experience profound healing and unlock our full potential.

Why Are Chakras Important?

Chakras are essential because they serve as gateways for the flow of energy throughout our entire being – physically, emotionally, and spiritually. Here's why they are so important:

1. **Energy Balance:** Chakras are responsible for regulating the flow of prana, or life force energy, throughout the body. When these energy centers are balanced and aligned, energy flows freely, promoting health and vitality. However, when chakras are blocked or imbalanced, it can lead to physical, emotional, and mental disturbances.

2. **Emotional Well-being:** Each chakra is associated with specific emotions and psychological functions. For example, the Heart Chakra governs love, compassion, and connection, while the Solar Plexus Chakra influences self-esteem and personal power. By working with the chakras, we can address emotional issues and cultivate greater emotional resilience and balance.

3. **Spiritual Growth:** Chakras are also gateways to higher consciousness and spiritual growth. The Crown Chakra, located at the top of the head, connects us to divine wisdom and universal consciousness. By balancing and activating the chakras, we can deepen our spiritual practice, expand our awareness, and experience states of profound spiritual awakening.

4. **Physical Health:** Imbalances in the chakras can manifest as physical ailments and health issues. For example, blockages in the Throat Chakra may result in communication difficulties or throat-related ailments, while imbalances in the Sacral Chakra can affect reproductive health and creativity. By addressing these imbalances through chakra work, we can support our overall physical health and well-being.

5. **Holistic Healing:** Chakra work offers a holistic approach to healing that addresses the root cause of issues rather than just treating symptoms. By addressing imbalances at the energetic level, we can promote healing on all levels – physical, emotional, mental, and spiritual. This holistic approach empowers us to take control of our health and well-being and facilitates deep and lasting transformation.

In summary, chakras are vital to our overall health, well-being, and spiritual evolution. By understanding and working with these energy centers, we can unlock our full potential, cultivate greater awareness, and live a life of balance, vitality, and inner harmony.

The Muladhara Chakra

Often referred to as the Root Chakra, is the foundational energy center located at the base of the spine. It serves as the root of our existence, symbolizing stability, security, and our connection to the physical world. Here's a closer look at the Muladhara Chakra:

1. **Location:** The Muladhara Chakra is located at the base of the spine, near the perineum, between the anus and the genitals. Its position at the lowest point of the spine anchors us to the earth and provides a sense of grounding and stability.

2. **Color and Element:** The Root Chakra is associated with the color red, symbolizing vitality, strength, and survival instincts. Its element is earth, representing solidity, security, and the physical world.

3. **Symbol:** The symbol of the Muladhara Chakra is a lotus flower with four petals, often depicted in shades of red. The lotus symbolizes purity and spiritual awakening, while the four petals represent the four aspects of consciousness: mind, intellect, consciousness, and ego.

4. **Energetic Significance:** The Muladhara Chakra governs our basic survival needs, including food, shelter, safety, and financial security. It is also associated with our primal instincts, such as fight-or-flight responses, and our sense of belonging and connection to the physical world.

5. **Imbalances:** When the Root Chakra is imbalanced or blocked, it can manifest as feelings of insecurity, fear, anxiety, or instability. Physical symptoms may include lower back pain, issues with the legs, feet, or spine, and digestive problems. Balancing the Muladhara Chakra is essential for establishing a strong foundation for overall well-being and personal growth.

6. **Balancing Techniques:** There are various techniques for balancing the Root Chakra, including yoga poses, meditation, breathwork, affirmations, and working with grounding crystals such as hematite or red jasper. Connecting with nature, practicing gratitude, and establishing healthy routines can also help restore balance to the Root Chakra.

In summary, the Muladhara Chakra is the foundation of our energetic system, providing stability, security, and a sense of connection to the physical world. By balancing and nurturing this vital energy center, we can establish a strong foundation for personal growth, empowerment, and overall well-being.

The Svadhishthana Chakra

Often referred to as the Sacral Chakra, is the second primary energy center in the human body. It is located in the lower abdomen, approximately two inches below the navel, and is associated with our emotions, creativity, and sexual energy. Let's explore the Svadhishthana Chakra in more detail:

1. **Location:** The Svadhishthana Chakra is situated in the lower abdomen, just below the navel. Its location corresponds to the sacral plexus, which is a network of nerves located in the pelvic area.

2. **Color and Element:** The Sacral Chakra is associated with the color orange, symbolizing warmth, creativity, and vitality. Its element is water, representing fluidity, adaptability, and emotional balance.

3. **Symbol:** The symbol of the Svadhishthana Chakra is a six-petaled lotus flower, often depicted in shades of orange. The lotus represents purity and spiritual awakening, while the six petals symbolize the six main qualities associated with this chakra: desire, pleasure, passion, creativity, abundance, and sexuality.

4.   **Energetic Significance:** The Svadhishthana Chakra governs our emotions, creativity, pleasure, and sensuality. It is associated with our ability to experience and express emotions, form healthy relationships, and tap into our creative potential. A balanced Sacral Chakra allows us to experience joy, passion, and intimacy in our lives.

5.   **Imbalances:** When the Sacral Chakra is imbalanced or blocked, it can manifest as emotional instability, low self-esteem, lack of creativity, and difficulty forming intimate relationships. Physical symptoms may include reproductive issues, lower back pain, and urinary problems.

6.   **Balancing Techniques:** There are various techniques for balancing the Sacral Chakra, including yoga poses, meditation, breathwork, journaling, and creative expression. Working with affirmations, visualization, and healing crystals such as carnelian or orange calcite can also help restore balance to the Svadhishthana Chakra.

By nurturing and balancing the Svadhishthana Chakra, we can cultivate a greater sense of emotional well-being, creativity, and pleasure in our lives. Embracing our emotions, honoring our desires, and tapping into our creative energy allows us to live authentically and experience life to its fullest.

The Manipura Chakra

Also known as the Solar Plexus Chakra, is the third primary energy center in the human body. It is located in the upper abdomen, just above the navel, and is associated with personal power, self-esteem, and willpower. Let's delve deeper into the Manipura Chakra:

1.   **Location:** The Manipura Chakra is situated in the upper abdomen, between the navel and the bottom of the rib cage. Its location corresponds to the solar plexus, a complex network of nerves located behind the stomach.

2. **Color and Element:** The Solar Plexus Chakra is associated with the color yellow, symbolizing energy, vitality, and intellect. Its element is fire, representing transformation, purification, and inner strength.

3. **Symbol:** The symbol of the Manipura Chakra is a ten-petaled lotus flower, often depicted in shades of yellow or gold. The lotus symbolizes purity and spiritual enlightenment, while the ten petals represent the ten qualities associated with this chakra: willpower, self-discipline, confidence, courage, determination, self-esteem, transformation, vitality, digestion, and metabolism.

4. **Energetic Significance:** The Manipura Chakra governs our sense of self, personal power, and autonomy. It is associated with our ability to assert ourselves, make decisions, and pursue our goals with confidence and determination. A balanced Solar Plexus Chakra empowers us to overcome obstacles, take risks, and assert our boundaries.

5. **Imbalances:** When the Solar Plexus Chakra is imbalanced or blocked, it can manifest as low self-esteem, lack of confidence, indecisiveness, and difficulty asserting oneself. Physical symptoms may include digestive issues, stomach ulcers, adrenal fatigue, and chronic fatigue syndrome.

6. **Balancing Techniques:** There are various techniques for balancing the Solar Plexus Chakra, including yoga poses, meditation, breathwork, visualization, and affirmations. Practicing self-care, setting healthy boundaries, and engaging in activities that boost self-confidence can also help restore balance to the Manipura Chakra.

By nurturing and balancing the Manipura Chakra, we can cultivate a greater sense of self-assurance, confidence, and personal power. Embracing our inner strength, honoring our authentic self, and trusting in our abilities allows us to navigate life's challenges with courage and resilience.

The Anahata Chakra

Also known as the Heart Chakra, is the fourth primary energy center in the human body. It is located at the center of the chest, near the heart, and is associated with love, compassion, and emotional well-being. Let's explore the Anahata Chakra in more detail:

1. **Location:** The Heart Chakra is situated in the center of the chest, at the level of the heart. Its location corresponds to the cardiac plexus, a network of nerves located behind the sternum.

2. **Color and Element:** The Heart Chakra is associated with the color green, symbolizing growth, healing, and harmony. In some traditions, it is also associated with the color pink, representing unconditional love and compassion. Its element is air, signifying openness, freedom, and connection.

3. **Symbol:** The symbol of the Anahata Chakra is a twelve-petaled lotus flower, often depicted in shades of green or pink. The lotus symbolizes purity and spiritual awakening, while the twelve petals represent the twelve qualities associated with this chakra: love, compassion, forgiveness, acceptance, empathy, gratitude, kindness, generosity, harmony, balance, peace, and interconnectedness.

4. **Energetic Significance:** The Heart Chakra governs our capacity to give and receive love, both to ourselves and others. It is the center of compassion, empathy, and emotional healing. A balanced Heart Chakra enables us to experience deep connections, foster harmonious relationships, and cultivate inner peace.

5. **Imbalances:** When the Heart Chakra is imbalanced or blocked, it can manifest as feelings of loneliness, isolation, resentment, or bitterness. Physical symptoms may include heart-related issues, such as high blood pressure, heart palpitations, or respiratory problems. Emotional wounds, such as grief, loss, or betrayal, can also impact the health of the Heart Chakra.

6. **Balancing Techniques:** There are various techniques for balancing the Heart Chakra, including heart-opening yoga poses, loving-kindness meditation, breathwork, and self-compassion practices. Cultivating gratitude, practicing forgiveness, and engaging in acts of kindness and service can also help restore balance to the Anahata Chakra.

By nurturing and balancing the Heart Chakra, we can cultivate a deeper sense of love, compassion, and connection in our lives. Opening our hearts to ourselves and others allows us to experience greater joy, fulfillment, and emotional well-being.

The Vishuddha Chakra

Also known as the Throat Chakra, is the fifth primary energy center in the human body. It is located in the throat region, near the thyroid gland, and is associated with communication, self-expression, and authenticity. Let's explore the Vishuddha Chakra in more detail:

1. **Location:** The Throat Chakra is situated in the region of the throat, near the Adam's apple. Its location corresponds to the cervical plexus, a network of nerves located in the neck.

2. **Color and Element:** The Vishuddha Chakra is associated with the color blue, symbolizing clarity, truth, and self-expression. Its element is ether, also known as akasha or space, representing spaciousness, expansiveness, and the infinite potential of communication.

3. **Symbol:** The symbol of the Vishuddha Chakra is a sixteen-petaled lotus flower, often depicted in shades of blue. The lotus symbolizes purity and spiritual transformation, while the sixteen petals represent the sixteen vowels of the Sanskrit alphabet, which are associated with the chakra's qualities.

4. **Energetic Significance:** The Throat Chakra governs our ability to communicate effectively and express ourselves authentically. It is the center of self-expression, creativity, and truth. A balanced Vishuddha Chakra enables us to speak our truth with confidence, listen actively, and express ourselves creatively through various forms of artistic expression.

5. **Imbalances:** When the Throat Chakra is imbalanced or blocked, it can manifest as difficulties in communication, such as speaking too much or too little, fear of public speaking, or feeling unheard or misunderstood. Physical symptoms may include sore throat, thyroid imbalances, or neck and shoulder tension. Emotional suppression, dishonesty, or unresolved conflicts can also impact the health of the Vishuddha Chakra.

6. **Balancing Techniques:** There are various techniques for balancing the Throat Chakra, including chanting, singing, mantra repetition, and throat-opening yoga poses. Journaling, creative writing, and engaging in conversations that honor your truth can also help activate and balance the Vishuddha Chakra. Practicing active listening and speaking with clarity and integrity are essential for nurturing the health of this energy center.

By harmonizing and balancing the Vishuddha Chakra, we can enhance our ability to express ourselves authentically, communicate with clarity and compassion, and forge deeper connections with others. Opening our throats allows us to speak our truth, share our creativity, and contribute to the world with authenticity and integrity.

The Ajna Chakra

Also known as the Third Eye Chakra, is the sixth primary energy center in the human body. Located in the center of the forehead, between the eyebrows, it is associated with intuition, insight, and inner wisdom. Let's delve into the Ajna Chakra in more detail:

1. **Location:** Positioned between the eyebrows, the Ajna Chakra corresponds to the pineal gland in the physical body. Its location symbolizes the seat of intuition and higher perception.

2. **Color and Element:** The Third Eye Chakra is often depicted as indigo or deep purple, representing inner vision, intuition, and spiritual insight. Its element is light, signifying illumination, clarity, and inner knowing.

3. **Symbol:** The symbol of the Ajna Chakra is a two-petaled lotus flower with an inverted triangle in the center. The lotus symbolizes purity and spiritual awakening, while the inverted triangle represents the merging of the physical and spiritual realms, as well as the union of feminine and masculine energies.

4. **Energetic Significance:** The Ajna Chakra governs our ability to perceive the unseen, trust our intuition, and access higher states of consciousness. It is the center of insight, imagination, and psychic awareness. A balanced Third Eye Chakra allows us to see beyond the limitations of the physical world and perceive the interconnectedness of all things.

5. **Imbalances:** When the Third Eye Chakra is imbalanced or blocked, it can manifest as difficulties in trusting one's intuition, feeling disconnected from one's inner guidance, or experiencing confusion and mental fog. Physical symptoms may include headaches, migraines, vision problems, or sleep disturbances. Overly rigid beliefs or excessive skepticism can also hinder the flow of energy in the Ajna Chakra.

6. **Balancing Techniques:** There are various practices to balance the Third Eye Chakra, including meditation, visualization, and mindfulness. Practices that stimulate the pineal gland, such as certain yoga asanas and pranayama techniques, can also help activate the Ajna Chakra. Spending time in nature, journaling, and working with symbols and archetypes are additional ways to nurture the health of this energy center.

By harmonizing and balancing the Ajna Chakra, we can deepen our intuition, expand our awareness, and access higher levels of consciousness. Opening our Third Eye allows us to perceive the world with greater clarity, insight, and spiritual understanding, leading to a deeper sense of purpose and alignment with our true selves.

The Sahasrara Chakra,

Also known as the Crown Chakra, is the seventh primary energy center in the human body, representing our connection to the divine and higher consciousness. Let's delve into the Sahasrara Chakra and explore its significance:

1. **Location:** The Sahasrara Chakra is situated at the crown of the head, above the top of the skull. It is often depicted as a thousand-petaled lotus flower, symbolizing its expansive and multi-dimensional nature.

2. **Color and Element:** The Sahasrara Chakra is associated with the color violet or white, representing purity, spirituality, and enlightenment. Its element is often considered to be consciousness itself, transcending the limitations of the physical realm.

3. **Symbol:** The symbol of the Sahasrara Chakra is a lotus with a thousand petals, which signifies the infinite potential and vastness of consciousness. The lotus blooms at the crown of the head, symbolizing the awakening of higher awareness and spiritual enlightenment.

4. **Energetic Significance:** The Crown Chakra serves as the gateway to higher consciousness and spiritual realization. It is the seat of divine connection, cosmic wisdom, and universal consciousness. When the Sahasrara Chakra is open and balanced, we experience a deep sense of unity with the universe, profound spiritual insight, and a profound understanding of our interconnectedness with all beings.

5. **Imbalances:** An imbalanced or blocked Sahasrara Chakra can lead to feelings of disconnection from the divine, spiritual apathy, and a lack of purpose or meaning in life. Physical manifestations of imbalance may include headaches, migraines, or neurological disorders. A closed Crown Chakra can also result in a rigid attachment to dogma, spiritual elitism, or an inability to integrate spiritual experiences into everyday life.

6. **Balancing Techniques:** Practices that help balance the Sahasrara Chakra include meditation, prayer, chanting, and contemplation. Connecting with nature, engaging in acts of service, and cultivating gratitude can also help open and activate the Crown Chakra. Crown-opening yoga poses, such as headstands or supported shoulder stands, can stimulate energy flow to this area.

By nurturing and balancing the Sahasrara Chakra, we can awaken to our highest potential, transcend the limitations of the ego, and experience a profound sense of unity with all of creation. Opening the crown allows us to tap into the infinite wisdom of the universe and experience the profound joy of spiritual realization.

Final Thought

Dear readers, as we conclude our journey through the realm of the 7 chakras, I hope you've found inspiration, insight, and perhaps even a touch of magic along the way. Exploring the intricate web of energy centers within ourselves can be a transformative experience, leading to greater self-awareness, balance, and inner harmony.

Remember, the journey of self-discovery is ongoing, and the wisdom of the chakras offers endless opportunities for growth and evolution. Whether you're just beginning to explore the world of energy healing or you're a seasoned practitioner, may the knowledge gleaned from this guide serve as a guiding light on your path.

As we bid adieu for now, I want to express my deepest gratitude for joining me on this journey. Your curiosity, dedication, and open-heartedness have made this exploration all the more enriching. May you carry the wisdom of the chakras with you in all that you do, and may your journey be filled with love, light, and boundless blessings.

Until we meet again, dear readers, I wish you all the best on your continued adventures. May your days be filled with joy, your hearts with peace, and your spirits with the ever-present glow of inner radiance. Farewell for now, and until next time, keep shining bright!

With warmest regards

Ellie Grace Rivers

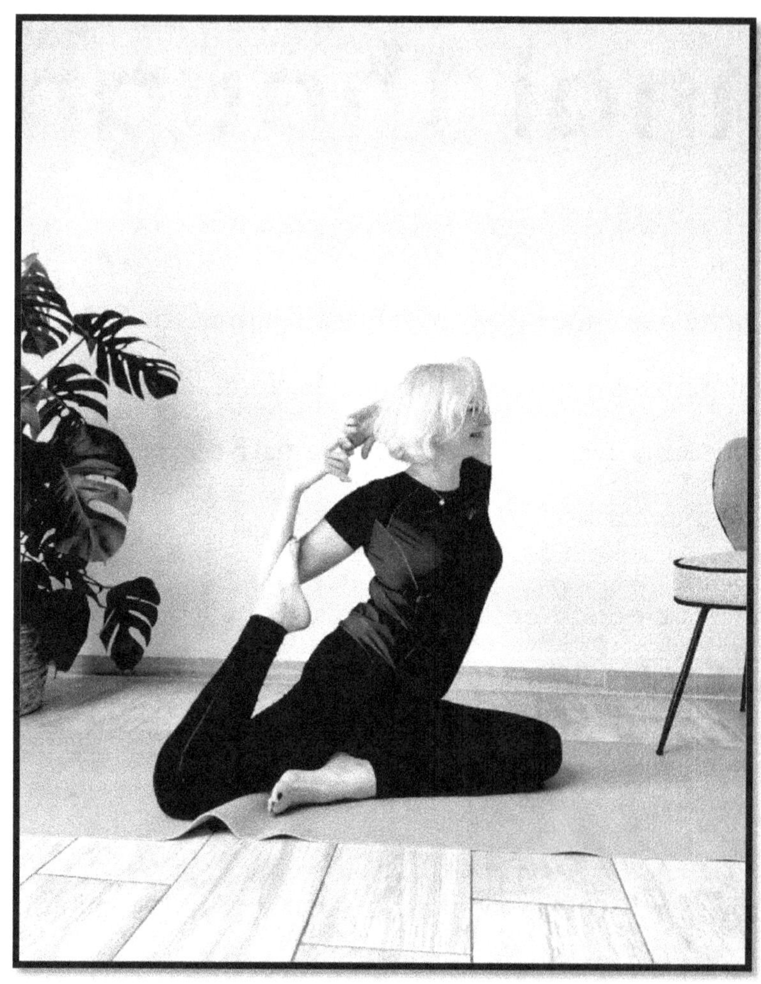